Emotional Eating

The Effective Guide for Intuitive Eating, without stick a strict diet and find the right motivation to build a successful future!

[Dr. John Zaradan]

Table of Contents

Emotional Eating Checklist

If you are fond of eating when you are full, or you like to eat whatever comes your way, there is a high probability that you succumb to emotional eating. One is said to have emotional appetite should there be a craving when there is no real hunger. Most time, you might not be able to differentiate emotional hunger from real hunger.

Kindly place a checklist if any of the following applies to you

- Food to me is a drug to tame emotions that are difficult to control like rage, sadness, frustration, joy, loneliness, helplessness, etc.
- Food helps relax my muscle in the presence of unpleasant body sensations such as muscle tension and nervousness
- I find comfort in eating
- When I am stressed, I eat
- When I feel powerless, I eat
- I eat for the excitement and pleasure of it
- Food is a tool to get rid of negative thought and calm my mind
- When I am powerless and paralyzed, I eat
- I don't really have a solid purpose or passion in life so I eat
- There is an emptiness in me and seems it can only be filled with food
- Food helps me forget the many regrets I have about my life
- Food is a reward to me
- Food is a punishment to me
- Food can be a weapon of rebel against someone or something
- Feeling satisfied brings a feeling of safety so I eat
- I hate sex, so I eat

- I am so occupied with food that it limits my progress in life

- I can only be satisfied with life when I take some of my favorite foods

You will benefit from reading this book if you have checked off one or more of the above. It is an indication that your eating habit has some emotional link to it.

Introduction

How seriously do you take your eating?

Have you ever considered that there is a possible connection between your emotions and your consumption of food?

There are a couple of other questions that are related to the above. Questions like; do you find it inevitable to eat only when you are anxious? And how do you feel when you are done eating? Do you notice any difference in the quantity of food that you consume when you are stressed and when you are happy?

The concept of emotional eating is not an alien topic, as we will see later in this book. We have all experienced it at one point in our lives. Both words are not new to us. But many are yet to come to the conclusion that our emotions have the tendency to trigger our consumption of food. You must have done this before, whether at your workplace or in your home or after having an intense discussion with your neighbor. If you have ever found yourself craving to satisfy your stomach amid emotional manifestations, then you could be considered as engaging in emotional eating.

Sadly, many people do not realize this or go to the extent of refuting the claim that it exists and that they cannot fall victim of emotional eating. Blindly, they consider their consumption of food at any point in time and any hour of the day as a result of hunger, which is entirely normal for every human. The reality is that emotional eating exists, and it can be experienced by men and women, young and old. But why should we conclude so?

Many a time, we always want to find comfort during emotional distress, to relieve ourselves off from the negative situation we are facing, and embrace solace outside that unwanted circumstance. Of course, it is good to be aware of your present situation and to create the intention of improving it. But what is not so good is allowing the awareness to trigger the unnecessary craving for food. This, sometimes, if not all the time, can develop into a bad habit and on the long run, affect our healthy lifestyle.

If emotional eating is not so fun, what are the possible consequences of doing it? Consider this simple illustration; we experience a lot every day, and our minds process what we exhibit as emotional reactions. If at every point in time that you feel depressed, stressed, or angry over a thing or situation, you grab something – whatever it is you can eat – and you consume it at that instant; what do you think happens? Your body reacts, and there is an immediate but temporal influx of energy. But does it solve the problem? No. you continue to feed your body with junks and foods even when you are not hungry. I bet you could figure out issues that could arise as a result of this. You would encounter the dangers of emotional eating in the course of reading this book.

Overcoming emotional eating is not as easy as many might consider it to be. This is so because we are not always conscious of falling for the triggers to control them. Also, our emotions initiate the act, so it will be a bit difficult to control our unnecessary appetites when we experience emotional outbreaks. For instance, how do you expect a person to control his urge for food when he is angry or stressed? What I am saying is, it is quite the work to overcome it.

I have often heard people saying that they seem not to be able to control the impulse to grab something to eat every time they are in one emotional state or the other. This is true to an extent. We all can fall under the control of our emotions some of the time so entirely that we become helpless in every other aspect of our lives. But one other fact that is worthy to note is that we can control our minds. And by taking control of our minds, we would be able to separate the craving for food from our emotions consciously.

How would you like to be free from emotional eating?

Emotional eating affects not only our health but also our lifestyle. This is why I have written this book. To serve as a guide to help cultivate your intuitive eating habit, to activate control of emotional triggers for unnecessary food consumption, and set you up on a spot-on diet plan. Food is essential in the body. We live on it and from it, and it is a factor to consider when planning our lives. So it is imperative that we have control over our food intake, especially in situations where we are not at all hungry.

This book will tell you how to build a successful life through controlled and healthy consumption of food. It contains the basics of emotional eating as well as practical tips that would help you to set up your life on a healthy living lifestyle. Having this book is a confirmation that you have decided to be mindful of emotional eating, its triggers, and that you have chosen the path to consciously control your reactions to emotional triggers and create a healthy living lifestyle plan for yourself to build a successful future.

Sail with me as we explore all that is to know about emotional eating. Do have a happy reading.

Chapter One: Emotional Eating Basics

Almost every conscious being has some idea about nutritional science. We all can recognize when it is time to eat and what we want to eat. Despite all our knowledge on nutrition, it is surprising to see that the internet continues to expand with various books on health and nutrition. Somehow, we keep learning new things.

One of the facts we should know about food is that we control what we eat, not the mouth nor the stomach. All they do is receive whatever we throw at them. Our food consumption might seem to involve the act of eating, but the reality is that our feelings are also very much involved.

What characterizes the concept of emotional eating can be described as the consumption of food, which is influenced by emotions, either negative or positive. In order words, our feelings can influence our decision making when it comes to eating. And this influence can be experienced at a fast pace.

This chapter will start with introducing what emotional eating is and how it is developed. Basically, all you need to know about emotional eating would be discussed here.

What Is Emotional Eating?

Does anxiety, anger, or sadness create an unquenchable urge to eat? Do you find comfort in eating after a heated argument with your coworker? When you are bored, do you keep opening the refrigerator, hoping to find something to fill your mouth with? If any of your answers to the above questions is yes, then you belong to the very many people that do the same thing as you in these raised circumstances. When you begin to use your emotions as an opportunity for you to satisfy your stomach, then there is a problem.

Simply, emotional eating is a condition whereby food is consumed as a result of the presence of specific emotional reactions. Emotions are what we feel while eating is an act of consuming food. Emotional eating is practiced because emotions are activated in our bodies. Many health practitioners and professional nutritionists consider the term to mean the habit of using food to be a form of relief, escape, or reward for something that we are experiencing at that point in time. For instance, emotional eating is eating when you feel upset, sad, angry, anxious, stressed, or embarrassed.

It has been concluded that emotional eaters see (emotional) eating as providing psychological nourishment rather than the biological purpose which food is created to serve. A quite shocking realization is that many people eat with their emotions and for emotional reasons, although some might deny being aware of it. In all cases, nonetheless, we all fall into emotional eating once in a while.

The routine practice of this act is an invitation to problems that might arise in almost every area of our lives. That is, when you continually use food to approach and deal with your emotions, you might end up having health and lifestyle issues that could keep you down for a long time. Rather than recognize their physical hunger and adequately satisfy their stomachs, emotional eaters conclude on killing their emotional hunger. The reality is that emotional eating cannot be the solution to the problem that activates the emotion, and as long as you try to use food consumption to control your feelings, you cannot have control of your diet and weight.

Some of the people who often partake in this ritual are well aware of its dangers, which we will be discussing later in this chapter. Still, they cannot help but rely on emotional eating to solve their emotional situations. Sadly, people who tend to be afraid to let go of emotional eating do this because they are not sure of any other way to manage their emotions. So, they continue to engage in eating as a substitute for facing their emotions and embracing the negative situation. Well, there are ways to face your fears, sadness, and stress, which also make the key to solving an emotional eating problem.

All You Need To Know About Emotional Eating

As a result of its popularity, scientists and psychologists continue to explore the concept, unraveling mysteries behind why people engage in emotionally eating. One prevalent fact is that many people who emotionally eat are aware of it and have good intentions to control and avoid it. But it just does not happen. Sometimes, you can end up digging into a bowl of cheese to calm your nerves and still feel the same level of anger. So why do you continue to do that despite the regret that embraces you aftermath the act? Here are interesting facts to know about emotional eating.

- Emotional Eating Can Work Like Drug

People who often emotionally eat are aware of the fact that their food consumption at that moment of their emotional experiences does not solve the situation but can only give momentary relief like drugs.

It is quite understandable that you might not be able to have your way with headspace meditation after the day's work, but visiting the food store is not the best idea either. Unfortunately, taking the fastest route to satisfy our tiredness and anxiety seems to be our best option. On this, this bestselling author Geneen Roth said, Even though many of you know that this is not the most effective way to handle your emotions, you just can't help it.

Like drug addiction, emotional eating can lead to feelings of shame and guilt. One can even end up trying to consume more to suppress the emotions. This is the cycle of emotional eating. If trying to suppress an emotion gives birth to another set of emotions, what do you think will happen? More eating, of course. This is, indeed, the emotional eating cycle.

- It Does Not Concern Food And Never Will

The words of the bestselling author Geneen are very important here. When you eat emotionally, she expressed: many people eat from compulsion that is not related with physical in any way. Rather, you eat because you are stressed and you feel like eating. This makes you use food as a tool to comfort yourself. Yet these emotions can be soothed in other reasonable ways.

The only problem is that you should never find the solution to your emotional trauma in a cup of creamy cheese. To find answers to your problems, you must face the source of the issue and not substitute that responsibility for eating food when your body does not require it.

Food is not the solution. It does not even concern it. But the urge to kill the stress or express our displeasure makes us see eating at that moment as an escape. People who cannot face their problems eventually take it out on food, which is an act that occurs almost every time.

- Your Quest For Comfort

Apart from the fact that we eat emotionally due to biological reasons. Do you also believe that emotional eating can be done to satisfy our physical body – for comfort? We must have experienced this when we were still in our mother's arms. She was always quick to quench our crying with breastfeeding. Also, consider the teacher rewarding the best student in your class with ice cream and the doctor handing out sweet to you every time you went for a checkup. It almost seems normal that our quest for comfort can lead to emotional eating.

It is also the case that emotional eating is seen to strengthen social relationships with others.

- Emotional Food Only Gives A Quick Fix

By now, you should know that emotional eating does not fix the emotion. Why is this so? It simple. Food consumption does not control your emotions. The only thing or otherwise, a machine that is capable of managing your emotions is your mind. And of course, food does not control your mind either. So, why would you consider eating your way of escape when you are stressed, bored, or sad? There are other effective methods to put your mind in control and manage your emotional responses. So why eating?

A study was conducted and reported in the Journal of Appetite. In the study, participants experiencing various emotional reactions were given chocolates to discover how emotional eating operates and how long it will heal them of their emotional traumas. In the report obtained, it was found that the length of time it took the participants to feel good before they return to their previous emotional state was three minutes. Just three minutes, it was not even up to one hour! The participants had only three minutes of freedom and calmness, and immediately the joy derived from the chocolates wore off, they were back at their state of distress.

It turns out you can only get three minutes of comfort and peace when you eat because of your emotions. It is surprising how short-lived the joy of emotional eating can be.

- Emotional Eating Is Mindless Eating

Just because it is emotional does not mean it involves your mind. Remember, in emotional eating, your mind is corrupted with negative feelings, which you have no control over and in constant agitation to get rid of them. Emotional eating does not allow you to be mindful of what you eat; neither are you concerned about the quality and quantity. In most cases, it is the quantity of the food you emotionally eat that is always unrecorded. You do not take notice of how much chips or cheese you consumed, and before you know it, you have eaten the whole bag or a full pint of ice cream. Because it is mindless eating, you are not able to regulate what you eat, and as such, it can lead to serious health complications. This is unlike satisfying physical hunger, where you are aware of what you are doing and taking notice of what you consume as food.

- There Is No Stomach For Emotional Hunger

It is not possible to store food in your brain. The only place scientifically proved to be a storehouse for food in the body is the stomach. And the work of the stomach is to house food when you are physically hungry or in case you are hungry. On the other hand. Your emotional hunger is not located in the stomach; neither is there a stomach for your emotional food. But it is the case that sometimes, we tend to feed our physical stomach with emotional food instead of using it to satisfy our physical hunger.

- Emotional Eating Does Not And Cannot Satisfy You

In emotional eating, you are not eating because you are hungry or because you would like to taste the new recipe. Instead, you eat because you are in an emotional state that you wish to get out of. If you are physically hungry, you will feed your stomach with what you are sure of to add nutrients to your body, and you will recognize it when your stomach can take no more. But in emotional eating, the fact is that you are never full.

Hunger does not exist in emotional eating. Or at least, not the kind of hunger that the body is supposed to experience. Emotional hunger does not exist, and if it does, it can be construed to be like outer space. And we all know that this space can never be filled. So, your emotional hunger is never satisfied. You keep wanting to eat more and more. On the long run, you keep consuming junks and overeating, which could end you up with serious health issues.

- Emotional Eating Is Circumstance-based.

Unlike physical hunger, which comes when the body has processed all the food in the stomach, and it is getting tired and hungry, emotional eating comes as a result of an emotional outbreak. For instance, the eating spree that is carried out after a heated argument in the board room, after a breakup or after a bet loss. So, emotional eating comes when you experience emotions, which usually show a terrible, negative, and unexpected occurrence.

As a result of emotional eating being situational, its hunger usually comes suddenly. A simple explanation for this is that the moment you experience the emotion, the hunger comes. It has been discovered that emotional hunger comes at an impulsive instant, usually urgent and irresistible.

- Emotional Foods Are Usually Specific

Emotional eating does not include eating healthy food like vegetables or organic foods. From a study, emotional eaters usually need junk food to satisfy their hunger. They are quick to choose sugary products over any other kind. This is why cake, ice cream, cheese, pizza, and related foods are commonly associated with emotional eating. To emotional eaters, it is all about sugar that will give an instant rush of energy and a positive vibe. Nothing else can do.

Statistics on Emotional Eating

Emotional eating is a common phenomenon, and everyone, at one point in their lives, has to do it. There is no shame in that. The only problem arises when emotional drinking develops into Binge Eating Disorder (BED), another fascinating topic related to emotional eating, which would be discussed later in this book. For emotional eating, below are some statistics given by the American Psychological Association (APA).

- 57 percent of American adults who are overweight have reported frequent emotional eating.
- It is discovered that 27 percent of American adults confessed that they eat to manage stress. Approximately one-third of the 27 percent confirmed that it had become a habit.
- About 33% of American adults who eat unhealthy foods or overeat said it distracts them from being stressed.
- Compared to men, women are more likely to report unhealthy eating habits resulting from stress.

Triggers of Emotional Eating

There are no unknown causes of emotional eating, only if we do not know them yet. According to facts discovered, emotional eating can be caused by both physical and psychological factors. Consider the following list of possible triggers of emotional eating.

- Emotions

Often, emotions are the primary triggers of emotional eating. These emotions include but not limited to, the following:

- o Stress
- o Sadness
- o Anxiety
- o Anger or agitation
- o Disappointment
- o Embarrassment
- o Pain
- o Tired
- o Broken or used

Positive emotions can also cause emotional eating, such as happiness, excitement, and feeling relieved. In essence, your emotions can cause hunger, which must be satisfied as soon as possible. When you succumb to this urge, and you finally grab a snack, you feel relieved and calm. The relief being momentary would cause you to continue eating because you do not want to leave that place of calmness and peace. Hence, you begin to overeat to stay in your comfort zone.

- Habits

Habits can also trigger emotional eating. If, at the end of school hours, you get home and are greeted with a pot of cookies every day, you might later develop that habit unconsciously and continue to eat even when you are not hungry. This develops into a mindless eating habit.

- Fatigue

When you are tired, particularly from doing something unpleasant or undertaking a difficult task, you are likely to start craving food unnecessarily. It is not important if you are physically tired or not, but when you are having trouble focusing or concentrating on the task, eating might seem to you the answer of whether you need to continue with the task or not.

- Boredom

Boredom is a widespread emotional eating trigger. When you have nothing to do or bored, eating becomes the only work left undone. For those who are associated with exciting and active lifestyles, if at any point they feel bored or have nothing to do, it will be hard for them to turn away from the opportunity of snacking. There would not be a better way to feel the void.

- External Influence

Group eating is an effortless way to overeat. The constant going out with your colleagues after the day's work to grab dinner or drinks, or as a reward for a productive day might develop into an emotional eating habit. It is easy to overeat when with a group of friends or family.

- For Pleasure

Well, some people find pleasure in eating whether they are hungry or not, and in any place they find themselves.

The continued existence of the above triggers, if left unaddressed, can develop into another form of unhealthy eating habit. This is an aggravated form of emotional eating. It is called Binge Eating, otherwise known as Compulsive Overeating or Compulsive Eating.

Signs of Emotional Eating

Many people, including a few emotional eaters, do not know they have the habit. I am often asked how to identify the warning signs of emotional eating. The truth is that it is not always easy to identify the symptoms. This is because many people do not want to agree that stress or sadness can make you need to eat. Below are signs you should take notice of in your eating habit. The presence of these signs is a signal that you have the habit of emotional eating.

- You always try to soothe your emotions by eating. Your body reacts subconsciously to the emotions you experience by craving food. This reaction is so unconscious that you might not even be aware of it. All you know is that you crave food anytime you are feeling sad, angry, lonely, bored, depressed, broken, among other emotions.

- You always eat whenever you are stressed. That is, you are quick to get hold of food when you have tasks to complete.

- The emotional hunger comes all of a sudden, and the need to eat becomes urgent and uncontrollable.

- You tend to find comfort in food despite knowing that they are junks, and too much of them could cause harm to your health. You cannot possibly give any reason why you always want to bury your hands in sugary products like cake, ice cream, cheese, chocolate, and cookies. Despite their low or non-existing nutritional value, you still find solace in them.

- You are having an eating spree. You cannot stop or control yourself from overeating. You eat when you are not hungry, and when you are, you keep eating even after you are full. Despite eating continuously, you still feel the urge to eat more because you can never satisfy the hunger.

• You cannot seem to be committed to your diet plan. You desire to lose weight, but you always fall short of completing the day's plan.

• You desire to have specific kinds of food and would not feel at ease until you have them. You can go miles to get them just because you need to satisfy that emotional hunger.

• You continue eating until you begin to experience physical discomforts, such as the inability to work with ease and stomach pain.

• You depend on food to feel happy and are delighted whenever you eat. You are emotionally dependent on food.

• After eating, you feel happy, tired, lonely, and lazy.

• After eating unhealthily or overeating, you begin to experience unpleasant emotions such as guilt, anxiety, shame, fear, and hurt.

Problems and Complications Of Emotional Eating

So you find comfort in taking a slice of the pie, and when you do, you escape from the stress. Three minutes later, you are back to that same emotion, and then you grab another pie. This continues even after your stomach is obvious to have filled. You continue to escape this emotion by eating to feel better. "This feels absolutely good, and I feel better," you say.

But what is the problem with this? It may look harmless and considered a common event that occurs in everyday life. But there is more to this than meet the eye, and you would be surprised when you find out.

Emotional eating should not be an habit that you should sustain. What you do not know is that your health and entire lifestyle will pay dearly, more than you ever bargained for. Apart from ultimately developing into Binge Drinking, which has implications of its own, consider the following problems that emotional eating can cause.

- The Emotions Still Exist

Emotions are possible triggers of emotional eating, but that does not mean that emotional eating can solve the problem that led to emotions.

Why do you experience negative and horrible emotions in the first place? What are their sources? Do you possibly think eating can solve the problems?

One ugly truth about emotional eating is that doing it will not address the problem. It does not even remove the emotions. According to the study, it only takes three minutes to enjoy solace, after which you are back the victim of that same emotion that made you eat unnecessarily in the first place.

- It Does Not Reveal The Reason For The Emotions

Emotional eating can only show the trigger, but it does not reveal the cause of the trigger; neither does it provides ways to solve it. If you dip your head inside a bucket of water, does the earth cease to exist? Absolutely no.

- You Just Dropped The Control

When you eat to fight off negative and horrible emotions and equip yourself to attract positive and good ones, you become emotionally subject to food. That is, you need food to feel good, to have that sense of peace, and to stay positive. Like drug addiction, you are addicted to food to get high, excited, and fulfilled.

In any instance, should you deny yourself of food, you will now to experience emotional discomfort. The craving for food to satisfy your emotional hunger has created a hole in your mind that can only be filled with food and more food. Unfortunately, this hole is never filled. So you have to continue the never-ending task of eating.

- Physical Implications

Emotional eating is mindless. It does concern itself with your physical (stomach) capacity. When you consume food to satisfy your emotional hunger "that does not exist," you are setting a trap for yourself that could affect your physiology. For instance:

  o Emotional eating is a fast path to gain weight. You will gain enough weight that will surprise you in a matter of time. Weight gain can, however, become traumatic because of the stigma that comes with it and especially if the person does not want to gain weight.

  o Emotional eating, which causes weight gain, can cause a decrease in physical appeal, creates poor body image, and eventually resulting in low self-esteem.

  o There is a high intake of cholesterol because of the kinds of food consumed. For instance, junk foods such as desserts, pies, chocolates, and chips contain plenty of fats. This, on the long run, can cause poorer health.

- Emotional Eating Is Abusing The Body

This is generally what emotional eating is doing to the body. Putting the body through unnecessary work. As a result, when you eat to satisfy your emotional hunger, your body weakens because it does not have to go through that work. There is an increase in digestion, processing of food, and weight of the body. All of these are unnecessary.

What happens when you overwork your body? You begin to experience digestion problems, inability to walk with ease, and eventually fatigue.

- The Emotional Eating Cycle

We already note that after eating emotionally, the emotions that made you eat still exist neither do the problems disappear. It is a three-minute safe haven before you come back to reality. But you cannot stay and face negative emotions, so you grab something to eat again, then enjoy the positivity for another three minutes. This keeps going on and on. You become stuck with the problem, the emotions, and the habit of eating.

Chapter Two: Emotional Eating And Food Addiction

Anybody can experience emotional eating, and this fact has made it be almost a conclusion that it is a normal way of life. Although every person is bound to do it sometimes, it is nonetheless not normal. To state the obvious, it is a bad engagement.

Chapter one of this book already talked about everything there is to know about emotional eating, so this chapter will take it a step further. We would explore certain concepts related to emotional eating. Emotional eating is terrible, but it can get worse. In chapter one, I mentioned binge drinking, which is one of the concepts we would be talking about in this chapter. The aggravated state of emotional eating is what develops into binge drinking. Also, there is what we call food addiction. These two concepts, binge eating, and food addiction would be exhaustively explained in this chapter, although emphasis would be laid more on food addiction.

The purpose of this is to let you be aware of the possibility that your emotional eating habit is still easy to control compared to the two above mentioned concepts. To put it more clearly, when emotional eating has continued for a period, and there is no conscious effort to deal with it, you would eventually find yourself in the binge eating and food addiction conditions.

Binge Eating

Binge eating is an unusual and excessive consumption of food. This can happen at any time, whether you are hungry or not. Perhaps you know someone or have found yourself at one time craving for food more than it is normal. Binge eating is characterized by eating food in large quantities, which is usually to be consumed within a short period. Typically, binge eating is a type of eating disorder, and we will consider the disorder now.

Do you have that one coworker that always orders more than he can contain? Or you have a kid nephew whose parent usually serve a mountain-full of the plate during lunchtime? Or you have a friend who is always shouting for more at every party? These are all expressions of binge drinking, which can become an eating disorder if not addressed.

Binge Eating Disorder (BED) is the most common type of eating disorder. It involves the chronic consumption of food within a period, usually to the state of discomfort. The disorder is known to be compulsive, overeating, or the consumption of food in a somewhat uncontrollable manner or unable to stop.

Statistics On Binge Eating Disorder

This disorder is common, and its prevalence has made health practitioners and professional nutritionists, including private researchers to conduct different researches and surveys to determine the extent of the disorder. Below are recorded statistics on Binge Eating Disorder.

- According to the reports from the Centers for Disease Control (CDC), approximately 2 percent of the American population is affected by Binge Eating Disorder.
- In a national survey conducted by the National Eating Disorders Associations (NEDA), about 2.8 million American adults are suffering from Binge Eating Disorder.
- According to National Eating Disorders Associations, men take 40 percent of the total number of people suffering from BED.
- 70 percent of people with BED are obese, according to the Binge Eating Disorder Association (BEDA).
- The rate of those affected by BED is tripled compared to Anorexia and Bulimia combined.
- Binge Eating Disorder is more prevalent than HIV, breast cancer, and schizophrenia.
- The age in which Binge Eating Disorder can begin to manifest is in the early 20s.
- The disorder is most common among women than in men.

Causes

There are no exact causes of BED yet, but it has been discovered that there is a variety of factors that could possibly contribute to the development of Binge Eating Disorder. Consider the following factors.

- Psychological factor

Depression has been easily linked to binge eating. Taking solace in eating as a means of coping or getting out of emotions such as low self-esteem, stress, and sadness is very common.

- Biological factor

Biological anomalies can also cause binge Eating Disorder. Irregularities in hormonal compositions or genetic mutations can be associated with compulsive overeating as well as Food Addiction (FA).

- Individual

Personal perception of the body can result in binge eating. Traumatic experiences, such as accident or abuse, tends to intensify the possibility of binge eating.

- Social and Cultural factor

This includes social pressure on weight, the media's comments on human bodies, and how culture regulates people's lives.

Symptoms

Binge Eating Disorder can manifest through a combination of symptoms that can be emotional or behavioral. But these symptoms might not easily be noticeable. The following are symptoms to watch out in Binge Eating Disorder.

- Experiencing binge eating at least once a week. This must have continued for three months or longer.
- Eating continuously, even when you are full.
- Not being able to control or stop what you eat.
- Saving food to consume them in secret.

- Eating plenty of food when no hungry.

- Eating in the usual way when in public but gobbling when not in open space.

- Never getting satisfied no matter the amount of food you consume.

- Experiencing a lack of sensation when bingeing.

<u>Complications Of Binge Eating Disorder (BED)</u>

The consequences of BED are many, and they range from emotional, social to physical dangers. Some of the complications include:

- Adverse emotional reactions, such as depression, anxiety, and guilt.
- Digestive difficulties.
- Pain in the muscle and joint.
- Sleeplessness.
- Type 2 Diabetes.
- Hypertension.
- Cardiovascular disease.
- Tiredness.
- Isolation.

Solving the Problem

Binge Eating disorder can become devastating, and in some cases, life-threatening. It is a case that should not be taken with levity. The following are simple tips that could help overcome Binge Eating Disorder:

- Do not skip meals.
- Do away with diet. It can be unhelpful sometimes and ultimately trigger binge eating occurrences.
- Be mindful of your body's reaction to eating, especially when you are satisfied.
- Consume more fiber.
- Drink plenty of water throughout the day.
- Plan your meal.
- Do not forget to eat breakfast.
- Get enough sleep.
- Exercise.
- Get medical help from professionals.

Having explained all there is to know about binge eating, let us now consider the concept of food addiction.

Food Addiction

Many people have argued that there is nothing like being a food addict. "Everybody likes food," they say. Everybody is indeed a fan of eating. Our very existence depends on food as a form of sustenance. So, everyone, at least in their right sense, would not consider food as an enemy.

Food is an essential requirement for our survival. It affects almost all aspects of our lives, which include physical, health, and emotional aspects. It improves our wellness. Apart from the life-sustaining benefits that food provides, it also serves as a source of enjoyment and satisfaction. As humans, we are able to draw gratification and happiness through smells, tastes, and mere seeing food on the table. We all experience that feeling the moment we hear the call "food is ready."

If food is not so much of something, we can do without, how then can it go wrong? Can we actually fall into the habit considered as food addiction? What is food addiction itself?

The Definition

Food addiction is a behavioral addiction. It could be referred to as compulsive overeating characterized by the frequent occurrence of binge eating. Binge eating, as already been explained, means the consumption of excessive quantity of food while experiencing an uncontrollable urge to continue. Food addiction at first features cravings for food. A person is not consciously aware of the cravings and eventually finds himself unable to either control the cravings or cope without satisfying them.

The term food addiction is a relatively new and controversial term. It has nonetheless sparked interests from many health professionals. Like drug addiction and alcohol use disorder, food addiction is characterized by compulsion and an uncontrollable impulse to eat. It can, therefore, be referred to as compulsive behavior. This compulsive behavior usually is a response to emotional reactions.

So, the answer to all the questions raised concerning food addiction is that it is a health issue, and people can be addicted to it. It can cause serious health issues if not addressed.

Foods That Are Associated With Food Addiction

People can be addicted to any and all kinds of food. But many concluded researches had identified foods that can be closely related to food addiction. These foods are considered problematic, and one can easily get addicted to them. These are foods that have a high level of sugar, fat, and starch compositions.

The following are examples of foods that fall under this category.

- Chocolate.
- Ice cream.
- Cookies.
- Fries.
- Cheese.
- Candy.
- Chips.
- pasta
- Bread, especially white bread.

Eating all the above is a regular daily function that is necessary to maintain our bodies and lives in general. We need to sustain our energy levels and ensure that the fundamental biological processes in our bodies, such as cell renewal and growth, are maintained. However, while we are bent on keeping ourselves alive and in good condition, we should also note that the foods we consume do not only affect our bodies. They also have psychological effects on our brains. Thus, unnecessary and excessive food consumption can result in mental problems.

Statistics On Food Addiction

Increasing realizations have suggested that a connecting pattern can be drawn between compulsive eating disorders and addictions due to the addictive features of hyper-palatable foods. Discovering the prevalence of food addiction is rare, but few recent studies have shown that food addictive symptoms could be found in children, adolescents, and adults. More extended researches have indicated that the prevalence of food addiction has an increasing rate in obese people. Although food addiction cannot be sufficient to account for the obesity epidemic. Equally, the symptoms and eventual occurrence of food addiction could be found in underweight, overweight, as well as individuals with average weight.

- The increasing number of scientific researches indicate that like drugs, food can also possess addictive qualities.

- Approximately 20 percent of those who are considered having a healthy weight, 30 percent of people who are overweight, and 50 percent of those who are obese have been discovered to be addicted to specific food combinations and the precise volume of food consumed.

- Animal studies have indicated that food addiction is characterized by an increase in levels of dopamine in the brain, which is also what is present in drug abuse. The dopamine levels activate the reward system that makes the user always want to come back.
- According to a study conducted by David Kessler, the United States house more than 70 million food addicts.
- Food addicts weigh heavy and have higher percentage body fats.
- Women are more likely to get affected by food addiction than men.

Studies and surveys on the prevalence of food addiction continue to be taken by various health bodies. Sooner, a clearer picture of how food addiction operates and its commonness would be revealed.

Symptoms Of Food Addiction

Food addiction can be easily identified because it features binge eating behaviors and a lack of control over food consumption. Also, the signs of food addiction can be emotional, physical, and social, as we will see now. Here are the signs to look out for in determining the existence of food addiction.

- Overeating Or Eating More Than Intended

It is the truth that we do not know how to stop picking the cookies. There is no such thing as "just a bite." We do not stop and can only do when there is nothing left. This symptom is very common with food addiction.

• Craving To Eat More After Feeling Full

It is very possible to get cravings after eating a nutritious sumptuous meal. It is common even, especially if you have not had such a meal for some time. Note that craving is not the same thing as hunger. Hunger is the urge to replenish your stomach, which is of necessity. Craving, on the other hand, is the urge to continue eating despite being full.

Getting cravings is common and might not mean that you have a food addiction. Food addiction sets in only when the cravings become recurring and uncontrollable. And it is always hard trying to suppress them. The cravings are not a call to satisfy your stomach or hunger. They are a call for pleasure and satisfaction as a result of the dopamine released in the brain.

• Binge Eating Or Compulsive Eating

If you eventually give in to thee cravings and you start eating, you might eat so much that the only time you realize what is happening is when you feel discomfort in your stomach. Eating disproportionately until the stomach is excessively stuffed is a sign of food addiction.

• Experiencing Guilt

Nobody likes to eat uncontrollably and end up having stomach discomfort or not being able to work properly. But when this happens, the emotions of guilt and sadness come in. The feelings of having done something terribly wrong and letting down are experienced.

Despite the short state of regret and being remorseful, the person ends up doing it again. This is the addiction at work. Like all other kinds of addiction like a drug, sex, alcohol, food addiction, never stops repeating itself. The pattern is always on repeat.

- Eating In Secret

People who can end up being food addicts often prefer to eat in secluded places. This is because the uncontrollable urge to eat, and the eventual continuous eating would make them feel ashamed in public places. So, in a bid to satisfy their emotional food desires, they find an enclosed setting.

Others symptoms of food addiction include:

- Self-induced vomiting as a result of the stomach being excessively full.
- Eating to control emotions.
- Setting up yourself with a food restriction plan.
- Compulsive exercise.
- Recurring digestive problems.
- Chronic fatigue, decrease in energy, and restlessness.
- Continued but failed attempts to stop or control overeating.

Complications of Food Addiction

The repercussions of food addiction can leave lasting effects in every area of your life. If left unchecked, it can ruin your health and, ultimately, your life. The impact of food addictions cut across the physical, social, and psychological facets. They include but not limited to, the following:

- Kidney or liver disease.

- Fatigue.

- Malnutrition.

- Obesity.

- Withdrawal from hobbies and interests that were once enjoyed.

- Stroke.

- Depression.

- Low self-esteem.

- Increased feelings of stress and anxiety.

- Panic attacks.

- Withdrawal from public places and social events.

- Sleeping problems.

- Underperformance at home or a place of work.

- Low sex drive.

- Digestive problems.

- Heart disease.

- Irritation.

- Feeling sad and hopeless.

- Headaches and body pains.

- Harmful weight gain.

- Self-inflicted punishment.

- Laziness and quickly getting tired.

Treatment Of Food Addiction

Consider the above-listed symptoms and effects of food addiction, if you think you are struggling with it or know someone who might be struggling with it, below are treatments that could help correct your eating addiction.

- Know The Issue

The first step to overcoming food addiction is realizing something is wrong. People often do not intervene in matters of addiction as long as it does not affect them in any way. So, taking a right and closer look at yourself is an excellent place to start. Check whether you are experiencing any biological, emotional, or psychological issue that is negatively affecting your health, production, and life. When you discover the problem and accept it as being an issue that must be solved, then you have successfully started on the path of overcoming food addiction.

- The Triggers

Know the "feel-good" foods and ensure to altogether avoid them. To do this, make a list of the foods you crave or binge on and make an intentional resolution to stop eating them. This is not always easy, but to overcome them, you must be ready to fight to the finish. In essence, avoid the triggers by all means.

- Change The Patterns

You have to change your routines in a way that you avoid the triggers. Do a careful analysis of what you do every day, the tasks you undertake, and the places you go that tend to cause you to overeat uncontrollably. Whatever it is, you need to change them or get them out completely.

- Meditation

Instead of engaging in food eating when you experience some emotional reactions, meditation could actually help. For instance, meditation may be used to relieve depression and stress.

- Seek Medical Help

Addiction sometimes requires that you have someone to talk to. Fighting addiction by oneself could prove unproductive, so it is essential to speak to someone about it. You can seek medical interventions, such as behavioral therapy and addiction groups.

Also, there are available changes that you need to make to help you treat and manage food addiction. They include:

- Taking organic foods rather than processed foods.
- Keeping out of caffeine consumption.
- Ensuring the three balanced meals a day.
- Taking time to cook at home.
- Getting enough sleep.
- Having an eating plan.
- Drinking plenty of water.
- Be conscious of the dangers of food addiction.

Unless you make conscious efforts, food addiction cannot be resolved. It is, therefore, imperative that you are intentional about overcoming food addiction.

Chapter Three: Why Food Education is Important

Food Education

Good nutrition extends one's life as it supports strength, versatility, endurance, hearing, vision, and psychological capacities. Eighty-seven percent of aged Americans have at least one chronic ailment that food education can help resolve, like chronic lung diseases, cancer, cardiac diseases, dementia, diabetes mellitus, hypertension, high blood cholesterol, osteoporosis, obesity and overweight, and the inability to succeed.

Nutrition education could be termed as any arrangement of learning experiences intended to encourage the voluntary selection of eating and other nourishment related practices helpful for wellbeing. It is a vital component of giving sustenance to older people. Nutritional education benefits people with arthritis, anxiety, and depression. It might diminish the danger of psychological decline in old adults and is very vital in overseeing numerous chronic diseases.

The Impact of Nutrition on Your Health

Unhealthy dietary patterns have added to the obesity plague in the U.S: around 33% of U.S. adults are obese, and roughly 17 percent (or 12.5 million) of youngsters and teenagers aged 2—19 years are overweight. Even for individuals with healthy weights, a lousy eating routine is related to significant wellbeing dangers that can lead to death. These incorporate cardiac illness, hypertension, type 2 diabetes, osteoporosis, and specific cancer types. By adopting savvy food routines, you can help shield yourself from these medical issues.

The factors for constant maladies in adults, such as hypertension and osteoporosis, are progressively observed in youths, usually a consequence of poor dietary patterns and expanded weight gain. Dietary propensities developed during adolescence usually stick around even in adulthood. Therefore educating kids on the right nutritional routines helps them even till death.

The connection between proper nutrition education and healthy weight diminished chronic ailment risk, and all-round wellbeing is too vital to be ignored. By learning how to eat healthily, you'll enrich your body with the necessary nutrients, and your body will surely thank you for it. Similarly to exercising, rolling out little changes in your eating regimen helps a lot, and it's simpler than you'd think. What you will learn what to eat and how to eat if you take your time to learn about nutrition; this will eventually improve your health.

Benefits of Healthy Eating

A healthy diet incorporates an assortment of fruits of various colors, good fats, lean proteins, whole grains, and starches. Healthy eating also implies dodging foods with high salt and sugar content.

Here we'll take a look at the top ten advantages of a healthful diet, and also the proof that backs them up.

Weight loss

There are numerous advantages to eating well, which you will learn through proper nutrition education.

Weight loss can lessen the danger of chronic diseases. An obese person is always at risk of the following conditions:

- Cardiac disease
- Non-insulin dependent diabetes mellitus
- Poor bone density
- Specific cancers

Vegetables and fruits contain lesser calories than most processed nourishments. An individual hoping to become fit ought to decrease their calorie consumption to basically what the body demands. To decide a person's calorie requirement, simply utilize the dietary guidelines distributed by the U.S government.

Keeping-up a proper eating routine free from prepared food can assist an individual with staying within their day to day limit without counting calories.

Fiber is one component of healthy eating routines that is very significant for overseeing weight. Plant-based nourishments possess dietary fiber aplenty, which manages hunger by making individuals feel more-full for longer.

In 2018, scientists discovered that nutrients rich in fiber and lean proteins brought about weight loss without having to check calories

Reduced Risk of Cancer

An unhealthful eating regimen can result in obesity. This could also lead to individual developing cancer.

In 2014, some researchers were able to prove that obesity added to an awful condition for individuals with cancer.

Be that as it may, taking fruits and vegetables can assist the fight against cancer.

In a different report from 2014, analysts discovered that eating fruits lessens the danger of cancer of the upper gastrointestinal tract. They also found that an eating regimen rich in vegetables, fruits, and fiber decreased the threat of colorectal cancer and that a regimen containing fiber reduces the danger of liver disease.

Numerous Phytochemicals found in fruits, vegetables, legumes, and nuts serve as antioxidants, which shield cells from harm that can cause disease. The beta-carotene, lycopene, and nutrients A, C, and E are a few examples of these antioxidants.

Tests done on people have been uncertain; however, lab and animal results have connected specific antioxidants to a lower incidence of free extreme harm related to cancer.

Diabetes management

Consuming a healthful diet will assist an individual with diabetes to:

- lose weight, whenever required

- manage blood glucose levels
- maintain blood pressure and cholesterol inside targeted ranges
- prevent or defer intricacies of diabetes

People diagnosed with diabetes should know that it is essential to reduce their consumption of nourishments with high sugar and salt content. Also, one should stay away from fried foods with high fats content.

Heart health and stroke prevention

Figures circulated in 2017, stated that 92.1 million individuals in America are suffering from at least one kind of heart-related malady.

As indicated by the Heart and Stroke Foundation of Canada, as much as 80% of instances of premature heart illness and stroke can be counteracted by a change in lifestyle, like, working-out more and dieting correctly.

There is some proof that vitamin E may avert blood clots, which can prompt cardiovascular failures. Below is a list of nourishments rich in vitamin E:

- Almonds
- Peanuts
- Hazelnuts
- Sunflower seeds
- Green vegetables

The connection between trans fats and heart-related sicknesses has been discovered by the medicinal community long ago.

If individual cuts-out trans fat from the eating routine, this will decrease their degree of low-density lipoprotein cholesterol. This sort of cholesterol causes plaque to gather in the arteries and can cause heart attack and stroke.

Lowering blood pressure can benefit the heart as well as restricting salt consumption to 1,500 milligrams daily.

Many processed and fast foods contain salt, and individual planning to bring down their blood pressure should not consume them.

Your kid's health

Kids adopt most of their health-related practices from the grown-ups in the environment; therefore, parents and guardians should pass on healthful eating routines.

Eating at home helps as well as. In 2018, analysts discovered that kids who consistently eat with their families ate more vegetables and less sugary nourishments than their companions who ate at the homeless.

What's more, kids who take part in planting and cooking at home might be bound to settle on healthful dietary and lifestyle decisions.

Healthy bones and teeth

A diet enriched with calcium and magnesium is essential for healthy bones and teeth. Keeping the bones sound is indispensable in counteracting osteoporosis and osteoarthritis down the road.

Below are foods high in calcium:

- Low-fat dairy products
- Broccoli
- Cauliflower
- Cabbage
- Canned fish with bones
- Tofu
- Legumes

Likewise, numerous grains and plant-based milk are rich in calcium.

Magnesium is copious in numerous nourishments, and the best ones are leafy green vegetables, nuts, whole grains, and seeds.

Improved Mood

New studies reveal a link between food and mood. In 2016, scientists discovered that food rich in glycemic load might result in higher manifestations of depression and exhaustion.

Food rich in glycemic load incorporates many refined carbohydrates, like, those in soda pops, cakes, white bread, and scones. Whole fruit, vegetables, and entire grains possess lesser glycemic load.

While a stimulating eating regimen might improve a person's overall mood, it is necessary for individuals dealing with depression to see they're doctors.

Improved memory

A stimulating eating routine might help against dementia and psychological decay. A study conducted in 2015 distinguished supplements and nourishments that prevent these antagonistic impacts. They are:

- Vitamin D, C, and E
- Omega-3 fatty fats
- Flavonoids and polyphenols
- Fish

The Mediterranean eating regimen fuses a large number of these supplements.

Improved gut health

The colon is loaded with naturally occurring microscopic organisms, which assume significant roles in metabolic processes.

Some specific strains of bacteria produce vitamins K and B, which colon utilizes. These strains also help to battle destructive viruses and bacteria.

Diets with low fiber and high sugar and fat can change the gut microbiome. This will heighten inflammation in the zone.

A diet fortified with vegetables, legumes, fruits, and whole grains gives a blend of prebiotics and probiotics that enable good microbes to flourish in the colon.

Fermented foods, like, yogurt, kimchi, and miso, are fortified with probiotics.

Fiber is prebiotic, and one can easily find it. Also, it is found in vegetables, grains, fruits, and legumes aplenty.

Fiber supports consistent bowel movements, which assists in curbing bowel cancer and diverticulitis.

Improved Night's Rest

Sleep apnea, among other factors, can affect sleep patterns.

Sleep apnea happens when the airways get blocked continuously as one sleeps. Risk factors are obesity, drinking liquor, and having a poor eating regimen.

Drinking less liquor and caffeine can result in better sleep, regardless of whether an individual has or doesn't have rest apnea.

Quick tips for a healthful diet

Trading soda pops for homegrown teas is a constructive change in an individual's eating regimen.

There are lots of little, positive approaches to improve the eating routine, like:

- swapping sodas for water and natural tea

- eating no meat for at least one day in seven days

- Making sure that produce accounts for 50% of every meal

- switching cow's milk for plant-based milk

- Consuming whole fruits as opposed to taking juices, which posses less fiber and regularly contains added sugar

- Cut-down on processed meats, which includes lots of salt and may heighten the danger of colon cancer

- Taking-in more of lean protein, which is present in eggs, tofu and fish

An individual may likewise profit from taking a cooking class, and figuring out how to include more vegetables into meals.

A specialist or dietitian can give tips on eating a healthful diet as well.

Chapter Four: The Relationship between Emotional Quotient and Emotional Eating

Emotional eating is the act of devouring vast amounts of food (for the most part, "comfort" or junk foods) because of emotions rather than hunger. Specialists disclose that 75 percent of overeating is brought about by feelings.

Emotional intelligence alludes to the capacity of an individual to oversee and control their feelings as well as that of others. As it were, they can impact the feelings of other individuals too. Emotional intelligence is a significant expertise in leadership. It is said to contain five fundamental components, which are – self-awareness, self-regulation, motivation, compassion, and social aptitudes.

The Relationship between Human Emotions and Eating Disorders: A Scientific Overview

There have been so many indications of a link between eating and emotions in the past. Different researchers have attempted to find the relationship between how human emotions are regulated through the nutrition they pick. Thankfully, the numerous researches have yielded wonderful insights.

From the studies, scientists found that there has been an unexpected decline in the part of the brain where our emotions are interpreted. This area, known as the Amygdala is responsible for understanding our feelings and also the feelings of those around us. It was found that the Amygdala is clouded by anxiety, which can arise from what we eat and how we eat.

The findings correlate with the problem of Alexithymia, which is a personality disorder of being unable to have emotions or feelings. A person suffering from this disease can neither describe his feelings, identity them nor differentiate emotions from body sensations. Studies on Alexithymia suggest that most eating disorders are linked to the disease. More than 70 percent of people suffering from this disease are either anorexic or bulimic (two major eating disorders). The study was easily proven since most Alexithymia patients do not respond to drugs or therapy sections.

Therefore, from the findings, there can be no way to distinguish between emotions and eating because Alexithymia is linked to a serious nutritional disorder that requires medical help. The simplest way to explain this link is through the concept of Emotional Intelligence. Emotional intelligence or EQ is the ability to control and express your emotions with other people.

A quick survey of the general populace reveals that people with low Emotional IQ are always having problems with nutritional choices. The study which focused on those with eating disorders shows that more than 90 percent of them have low EQ and it had nothing to do with gender, age or physical attribute.

There are five components of Emotional Intelligence, and this includes Mindfulness, Self-control, Interpersonal Skills, Optimism, and Empathy. Psychologists have found that most people with eating problems are suffering from one or more of these components. The ways we eat and how we eat can be controlled by any of these factors and hence, affect our emotions.

More studies are required to build on this research. However, in conclusion, psychologists maintained that if people can improve on the five components of Emotional Intelligence, they will be able to resolve their eating disorders to a large extent.

Food Cravings: What does it Mean?

Humans crave certain nourishments because of the presence of some acids like amino acids and other types of catalysts. They are responsible for stimulating the body or calm your cerebral chemicals. Considering the case of somebody who's fatigued or burnt-out, they may reach out for cheese or soda to regain lost energy instantly. Most times, if people are frightful, depressed, or feeling forlorn, they may begin longing for the calming effects of foods similar to dessert.

Diets that are high in fats are more enjoyable as different foods fulfill our distinctive emotional needs.

Doreen Virtue researched dietary issues and the mental issues that cause food cravings and in the process, discovered a rundown of food concerning their emotions. According to her, emotional problems identified with food cravings are categorized into specific classes.

Four emotions make-up the central part of emotional overeating: these are

- Fear,
- Anger,
- Tension, and
- Shame

It can be used with the acronym FATS. Fear is an important and necessary part of the FATS emotions; all the others originated from it. We feel furious because we are scared of loosing something or someone so dear to us; tension comes to us since we fear trusting or as a result of losing the path meant for us; Shame also come when we fear and feel we aren't good enough.

If the emotional problems you face are unattended-to, your cravings will stay, and if the emotional problems change, so will your relationship with food as well. There might be some physicality to why some people have inordinate relationship with food. In case you lack minerals or nutrients, or you have imbalanced eating routines, you will hunger for specific foods. When the physical facet of your cravings is resolved, you're left with the emotional.

Confront your emotions. If you don't confront them, your yearnings will stay.

If your yearnings appear to be directed towards diets with high fat, it's probably because of some insecurity you're attempting to load up with fat.

The best course of action for dealing with bad and unhelpful craving is to resolve the issue from its root. Even little moves towards fixing any issue in your workplace or in your private life can lessen food cravings. Our dispositions influence our eating pattern, but so does our eating pattern on our mood.

This epitomizes the saying, "you are what you eat," particularly in connection to food and how we feel, in other words, mood. In any case, if you're on a balanced diet, you're bound to feel more at ease and generally better.

Ways Your Food Intake Can Affect Your Mood

Your dieting is irregular. Not expending the required calories can prompt issues like feeling foggy, worn out and fatigue.

You are removing or holding back on fundamental nutrition types, which the body requires to refuel and produce serotonin, which is the feel-good chemical of the mind.

You are overlooking fundamental nutrients and minerals. This leads to a lack of concentration, depression and constant fatigue.

Your body is not getting sufficient omega-3 fatty acids, which have been reported to reduce depression.

You're consuming processed foods in large quantities. This might result in a bigger waistline, feeling drowsy and conceivably lead to insulin imbalance and aggravation when taken too much.

Insulin levels: certain processed foods, particularly those with a lot of added sugars, may result in volatile insulin levels which bring about constant hunger.

Aggravation: Chronic irritation can be an aftereffect of a diet that incorporates a lot of manufactured and processed food. This prompts heightened degrees of C-receptive protein, which is related to the dangers of mental distress and misery.

Ways to Improve Your Mood through Food

Fill your plate with good-mood enabling diets by consuming a rainbow of fruits and veggies.

Eat more organic foods than processed ones. For instance, pineapple juice is processed and not as close to life as a pineapple fruit.

Consume more of diets like eggs, fish, legumes, and leafy green veggies as they are rich in dopamine.

Increments in the consumption of omega-3 fatty acids found in fish, flaxseed, and walnuts, can assist to battle depression.

Take more magnesium-rich foods, which aide sleep, like almonds, spinach, pumpkin seeds, and sunflower seeds.

Cut down on added sugars. Take fruits instead of treats sweetened with sugar.

Check your body's vitamin D levels. A low level of this nutrient is related to mood and depression issues. Vitamin D is contained in fatty fish, egg yolks, and liver.

Most metabolic issues originate from the emotion. It is known that the feeling impacts our body system as they are connected on a deeper than surface level.

For instance, stress adds to a variety of diseases, namely HBP (high blood pressure) cardiovascular issues and also metabolic issues.

How to Practice Emotional Intelligence When Eating

If you are only being too careful about what you're eating, you are only focusing on just half the idea. Watching what you eat is, for most people, very convenient to do since our society is continually centered on the type of food we consume. So we assume, "It was just about foods, so if I avoid certain foods or if I include certain foods, then I'll be good." But no one thinks at the possibility that if I'm very nervous about taking gluten out, my anxiety could potentially become a significant contributing factor for why I'm more definitely sensitive to gluten. With a thought like that, you are just aggravating the situation rather than emerging out of your dilemma.

The actual mechanism of eating is closely linked to our digestive health and physical health as a whole. Being mindful of what you eat, which means paying attention to how we eat, has so many physical and emotional advantages.

Rest after eating

Make out some time to rest and frequently meditate, most especially, if you usually eat up to three times each day. Stay calm, and try not to get distracted by another meal.

Eat with friends

The world today has deviated from taking suppers together. We eat in our vehicle; we eat in a hurry or decide to be separated from everyone else. In some modern families, the mother will send a message from the kitchen, and the dad and the youngsters will run from their separate rooms, get nourishment, and return to their particular places once more. It's essential to eat together as it helps people become self-aware of what they eat.

Connect with people when eating

When eating with friends or family, be connected with them by holding hands before eating. For reasons unknown, when we clasp hands, when we reach other people, our pressure reaction goes down. We are much relaxed and calmer. Since, as it were, you're telling your body: "I'm at home, I'm sheltered." Humans are natural herd. We grew up with the people in our society. Our subconscious mind reminds us that if we are with our clan, we're protected, but if we are without anyone else in the Savanna, we may be in threat. Thus, being in a gathering creates a sense of harmony. Along these lines, you clasp hands, and your feeling of anxiety goes down, which assists with the whole procedure of digestion.

Eating together really shields us from depressive thoughts, as well. There's a lot of information that supports that the leading cause behind misery is an absence of association. It can be seen when individuals feel desolate, detached, and not part of the network, which is a significant trigger for depression. Eating together and doing this now and then can serve as a neurochemical marker that discloses to you that I am presently in the network, I am currently protected, and I am presently cherished because oxytocin is being discharged.

Don't Rush Your Food

Relax and take a look at your food before devouring it. Look at the menu admiringly. Have some appreciation for the way that it's there. Look at the colors and the shapes. Take it in with every one of your faculties. There's now affiliation beginning just from seeing it. This makes you salivate, and salivation starts this entire procedure of absorption before you have even taken a piece from the food.

The amylase compound in your salivation prepares to transform starch into sugar, which causes you to make the most of your nourishment more. Take your first nibble, and you eat gradually. How that the flavor particles impart to your cerebrum is through the synaptic associations on your tongue on your taste buds. And this works best when wet, just like electric light. So when you eat gradually, there's sufficient salivation in your tongue that those markers can impart successfully. Also, you have significantly more flavor and sensation.

Also, this makes you satisfied quicker because you have had a great deal of flavor and taste. Also, ensure that you chew properly.

Don't Eat too Much

Stop taking too much food than necessary. Just take 60 percent of the food you can. That way, the stomach can blend the stomach related liquids appropriately after eating. This process is known as Peristalsis: the way your stomach stirs and needs to do this wave-like movement where it pounds stomach acids through the nourishment. If your stomach is genuinely filled after you have over-ate, then there will be no space in the stomach for blending the food. But, if you chew your nourishment well and don't overeat, it consumes and disintegrates rapidly. You don't have a bump in your stomach since it doesn't get foul while it's staying there. Keep in mind that each time you eat is a chance to support your body.

Breathe after eating

Breathing deeply after eating is so significant in consuming our fats. Humans are of complex carbons. Carbon with oxygen becomes carbon dioxide or carbon monoxide. If you have an outdoor fire, for instance, you're not going to get a decent fire if the pit fire is stifled. Toward the end, you will have vast coals left. But, if you have a decent oxygen stream, you have extremely clean fumes and an excellent flame. This creates more energy, and fine white ash left; it is similar to the way we consume our food. You need an appropriate oxygen supply to have enough accessible energy and avoid plenty of grimy fumes.

Smile

Smiling or laughing after eating is stunning, as well. You have heard the famous saying that laughter is "the best medication." It is. You can make a healthy joke or watch a comedy. Be filled with joy; it produces energy for healing. Incorporate this to be a piece of your meal, as well.

How you eat is as important as what you eat regardless of whether your objective with nourishment is to get more fitness, have more vitality, or ease uncomfortable indications. Focusing on the feelings behind your eating designs combined with careful eating practices could be only the ticket you have to arrive at your objectives in a reliable and manageable manner.

Chapter Five: Setting Limits and Resisting the Temptation to Eat

The only way to deal with emotional eating is through self control, and there are some practices that will make you achieve this easily. However, it is important to note some eating disorders that are psychological. This way, you can diagnose yourself and deal with it objectively.

Understanding Eating Disorders

Eating disorders are a variety of psychological states that lead to the development of poor eating habits. People with this disorder can start with a diet, body weight, or body shape addiction.

Eating disorders can lead to serious adverse health effects if it gets out of hand. It can result in the death of a person who did not detect it early.

Someone with eating disorders may have signs of various kinds. Some of them are severe food deprivation, binge eating, or purging habits such as vomiting or excessive exercising.

Eating disorders can be seen in all humans of any sex or age, but they are frequently seen in teenagers and young ladies. Yes, close to 13 percent of young people can experience at least one eating disorder.

What is the Cause of Eating Disorder?

Researchers say that a number of factors can cause these disorders. Heredity is one of such.

Twin and adoption research involving twins switched at birth and raised by different families has revealed some proof of inherited eating disorders. Generally speaking, this type of analysis has revealed that if one sibling has an eating disorder, the other has an approximate 50 percent chance of developing one as well.

A person's personality is also one of the causes. Neuroticism, perfectionism, and impulsivity are three character traits that are sometimes associated with an increased risk of developing an eating disorder.

Certain possible causes include perceived peer pressure to slim down social biases, and social media exposure supporting these values.

In addition, societies that have not been subjected to Western values show less risk of some eating disorders. Yet few people end up creating an eating disorder in several nations. Therefore, a combination of factors is likely to cause them.

Researchers have recently suggested that changes in brain development and physiology may also play a role in eating disorders.

Also, varying factors that can result in the rise of eating disorders are serotonin and dopamine levels in the brain.

Nonetheless, further studies are necessary before it is possible to draw definitive conclusions.

Types of Eating Disorders

Anorexia Nervosa

The most popular eating disorder is undoubtedly the anorexia nervosa. Throughout puberty or early twenties, it typically progresses and usually affects more females than males. Anorexics commonly see themselves as being obese, even if they are seriously lean. They prefer to control their appearance regularly, avoid eating other food types and greatly limit their calories.

Signs and symptoms of this disorder include:

- becoming substantially underweight compared to people of similar stature and size
- extremely small eating habits
- extreme fear of getting fat or constant habits to prevent weight gain while being super skinny
- the relentless pursuit of slimness and inability to keep a healthy weight
- the strong influence of body mass or expected weight on self-esteem
- A skewed view of the body, including rejection of being too skinny

This eating disorder can sometimes be attributed to signs of neurotic-compulsive. For example, most persons with anorexia are often concerned with food, and some may be incessantly collecting recipes or hoarding food.

These people may also have trouble eating outside and have a keen desire to control their surroundings, reducing their ability to be relaxed.

Anorexia can be divided into two variants— the type of that won't eat and the type that overeats and vomiting.

People with the restrictive form lose weight by diet, abstinence, or excessive exercise.

People with the form of binge eating and vomiting can binge on large quantities of food or take very little. In each of these cases, after feeding, they quickly use up the food through excess exercise, vomiting, consuming laxatives, or diuretics.

Anorexia can be detrimental to human health. Over the years, people who live with it may develop bone thinning, infertility damaged hair and nails, and the development of a layer of fine hair in their bodies. When the case becomes serious, heart, brain, or multi-organ, damage and death may occur.

Bulimia Nervosa

Another popular eating disorder is bulimia compulsive overeating.

Like anorexia, this eating disorder occurs mostly in adolescence and early twenties. Also, it seems to be less common among males than females.

Within a specific time frame, people with bulimia often eat exceptionally large quantities of food.

The eating goes on until the individual gets completely filled. The person generally feels throughout a binge that they simply cannot stop eating or regulate the amount of food they take.

The uncontrollable bouts of food can occur with any item on the menu, but most frequently with foods that would naturally be avoided by the person.

People with bulimia then try to vomit what they eat in order to make up for the food consumed and ease the inconvenience of the gut.

Compulsory nausea, fasting, diet pills, diuretics, enemas, and increased exercise are popular purging habits practiced by people with bulimia.

Signs may seem very close to that of anorexia nervosa overeating or purging variants. People with bulimia, however, tend to keep a reasonably normal weight instead of becoming thin.

Popular bulimia nervous signs include:

- Recurring incidents of overeating with a sense of lack in self-control
- repeated instances of unhealthy purging habits to avoid obesity
- self-esteem unduly influenced by body type and weight
- fear of obesity, even after having normal body weight.

Bulimia's adverse effects can include irritated and sore throat, enlarged salivary glands, broken enamel, cavities, stomach problems, intestinal pain, severe dehydration, and hormonal disorders.

Bulimia can produce a disparity of electrolyte concentrations, such as sodium, potassium, and calcium, in serious conditions; this can cause severe medical issues.

Individuals with bulimia nervosa eat huge amounts of food in short durations, then vomit. They are afraid to gain weight even though they are at a normal weight.

Binge Eating Disorder

Binge eating disorder, particularly in Americans, is considered to be one of the most prevalent eating disorders.

This eating disorder usually starts in puberty and young adulthood, even though it may grow afterward.

People with this condition have bulimia-like signs or binge eating anorexia.

For example, in fairly brief periods of time, binge-eaters normally eat excessively large quantities of food and experience a lack of discipline throughout their eating.

Those with food addiction do not reduce calories or use purging techniques to adjust their binges; they don't force nausea or perform excessive exercise.

Signs that are common to binge-eaters include:

- taking large quantities of food quickly, secretly and unpleasantly, even when they are not feeling hungry

- feeling uncontrolled throughout binge eating episodes
- moods of discomfort, such as embarrassment, disgust, or remorse, when worrying about binge eating behavior
- no use of purging habits, such as calorie restriction, vomiting; to make up for their excessive eating behavior.

Individuals with binge eating conditions are often obese and fat. This may increase their chances of excess weight-related medical problems, such as cardiovascular disease, strokes, and type 2 diabetes.

Individuals with binge eating disorder devour so much food in short periods of time on a daily and uncontrollable basis. They do not try to vomit as opposed to Anorexic and Bulimic people.

Pica Disorder

Pica is also an eating problem that involves feeding on non-food items.

People with pica enjoy non-food substances like ice, dust, water, chalk, soap, paper, skin, fabric, fur, pebbles, washing powder, or cornstarch.

Pica can exist in adults, teenagers, and young adults alike. That being said, this condition is most commonly seen in kids, pregnant women, and mentally disabled people.

People with pica may have a heightened risk of poisoning, diseases, gut wounds, and abnormalities in food. Pica may be life threatening based on the substances the person is eating.

Even so, consuming non-food substances should not be a standard practice of the culture or faith of anyone to be regarded pica. Moreover, it must not be regarded by colleagues of the person suffering from this disorder as a publicly acceptable action.

Rumination Disorder

Another eating disorder known as the rumination disorder has just been recently identified.

This is a disorder in which an individual regurgitates their earlier chewed and ingested food, re-chews this, and can either re-swallows it or vomits it out.

Usually, this behavior happens after a meal during the first 30 minutes. This behavior is voluntary, unlike medical issues such as colic.

This condition can progress during adolescence, infancy, or maturity. This can be seen to rise in children between the ages of three to twelve months and often stops by itself. Therapy is generally required for children and adults with the disorder to overcome it.

Rumination syndrome can cause weight loss and extreme malnourishment if not sorted in an infant. Adults with such a disorder, particularly those who do this in public, may limit the amount of food they eat. This can cause weight loss and thinness.

ARFID

Avoiding / Restrictive Food Intake Disorder(ARFID) is a new title for an old eating disorder.

The word replaces what was regarded as infancy and early childhood feeding disorder, a treatment that was specifically created for kids below the age of seven.

Although ARFID typically emerges during nursery or teen years, it may linger as they grow older. However, it is common among people of both genders.

People with this condition report feeding upset either due to lack of feeding desire or disdain for certain odors, flavors, colors, patterns, or temperatures.

ARFID's signs and symptoms involve:

- neglect or reduction of food intake which keeps an individual from consuming enough calories or nutrition
- dietary habits that conflict with regular social activities, such as eating with others
- losing weight or poor age and height development
- Deficiency in nutrients or dependency on vitamins or tube feeding.

However, ARFID does not involve food refusal or prohibitiondue to the lack of food supply or religious and cultural traditions.

Other Disorders

There are also less widespread eating disorders in addition to ones written earlier. These typically fall in one of three classifications:

Purging disorder: people with purging disorder always use purging activities such as throwing up, laxative, diuretic, or extreme exercise to maintain their weight or size. They're not bingeing, though.

Eating at night: People with this condition mostly eat inappropriately after waking up from sleep.

Specific feeding disorders: Although not included in the DSM-5, it encompasses any other disorders with health problems related to those of an eating disorder, although not outside of the latter classifications.

Orthorexia is one of the specific eating disorders. Although frequently stated in media and research reports, the current DSM (Diagnostic and Statistical Manual of Mental Disorders) has yet to identify orthorexia as a distinct eating disorder.

Individuals with orthorexia tend to focus on healthy eating to the degree that interferes with their daily lives.

For example, the person affected can exclude whole food groups in fear of being unhealthy. It can cause malnutrition, severe weight loss, out - of-home eating problems, and emotional distress.

People with orthorexia rarely focus on weight loss. Actually, their self-worth, personality or happiness depends on how well they are performing

The first two disorders are not well known at the moment. The class OSFED covers all eating disorders that do not fall into another category, such as orthorexia.

In conclusion, the above definitions are meant to provide a better understanding of and dispel myths about the most common eating disorders. Eating disorders are symptoms of mental health that typically need treatment. If left untreated, they can also damage the body.

Self-Control in Eating

Now that you have diagnosed if you have an emotional eating disorder, how can you treat it personally? Self-control

Self-control is a battle for some individuals, particularly with regard to nourishment. Eating a lot in one sitting or taking in such a large number of calories for the duration of the day are regular propensities that can be difficult to break.

After some time, eating an excessive amount of nourishment can quickly make you obese and put you in danger of ceaseless infections like diabetes and coronary illness. In addition, it can keep you away from arriving at your wellbeing and health objectives and may adversely affect your passionate prosperity.

In spite of the fact that breaking the cycle of gorging can be trying, there are approaches to kick this undesirable propensity for good.

Here are successful approaches to quit excessive eating.

Dispose of Distractions

Regardless of whether it's working through lunch before your laptop or noshing on chips while you get up to speed with your preferred network show, eating while diverted is a typical event for a great many people.

While this habit may appear to be innocuous, it might be making you over indulge.

A survey of 24 considers found that being occupied during a feast drove individuals to expend more calories at that supper. It likewise made them eat more nourishment later in the day contrasted with individuals who focused on their nourishment while eating.

Attempt to kill or take care of potential interruptions like telephones, PCs, and magazines so you can focus on your supper. It will assist you with eating less and stop indulging.

Know Your Weaknesses

Pinpointing which nourishments you have an especially hard time restricting can assist you with diminishing your odds of excessive emotional eating.

For instance, if you have a propensity for eating an enormous bowl of frozen yogurt consistently, quit keeping dessert in your cooler.

Planning sound choices like a cut apple with nutty spread, hummus, and veggies, or custom made trail blend can assist you with settling on better decisions when you are craving for a treat.

Another accommodating tip is to keep unfortunate nibble nourishments like chips, treats, and french fries far out with the goal that you aren't enticed to get a bunch each time you stroll past.

Distinguish the undesirable nourishments you can't help it. Keep them out of your home or out of sight and make sound choices effectively available.

Try not to Ban All Your Favorite Foods

Prohibitive eating designs that cut out a large number of your preferred nourishments may make you feel denied and drive you to binge on illegal treats.

Diets that focus on entire, natural nourishments are in every case best, yet preparing for a periodic treat is alive and well.

Swearing that you will never have a scoop of frozen yogurt, cut of pizza, or bit of chocolate again isn't practical for the vast majority.

Rather, center on furnishing your body with, for the most part, sound, nutritious nourishment while additionally giving yourself the opportunity to appreciate a treat to a great extent genuinely.

Eating designs that are too prohibitive may drive you to binge. The way in to a maintainable, solid eating regimen is to focus on eating entire, natural nourishments more often than not while permitting yourself a treat to a great extent.

Try Volumetrics Out

Volumetrics is a method for feeding that is based on topping off with low-calorie, high-fiber nourishments like vegetables that do not contain starch. Devouring nourishments that are low in calories and high in fiber and water before suppers can assist you with feeling full so you aren't enticed to indulge.

Instances of volumetrics-accommodating nourishments incorporate grapefruit, plate of mixed greens, broccoli, beans, tomatoes and low-sodium juices. Eating an enormous plate of mixed greens or a bowl of low-sodium, juices based soup before lunch and supper might be a viable method to counteract gorging.

Utilize the volumetrics strategy for eating: top off on solid, low-calorie, high-fiber nourishments to assist you with feeling full. You'll be less inclined to enjoy on unfortunate nourishments.

Abstain from Eating From Containers

Eating chips out of the pack, frozen yogurt out of the container or takeout directly from the case can lead you to devour more nourishment than you need.

Rather, divide out a solitary serving size on a plate or in a bowl to help control the quantity of calories you are expending.

To prepare your eye, give estimating a shot serving sizes for possibly 14 days until you comprehend what an ordinary segment ought to resemble.

Rather than eating nourishment directly from the bundle, partition it into a dish. Give estimating a shot fitting serving sizes to help train your eye to distinguish how a lot of nourishment is directly for you.

Decrease Stress

Stress can prompt you to eat excessively, so it's essential to discover approaches to lessen the measure of worry in your life.

Incessant stress drives up levels of cortisol, a hormone that expands hunger. Studies have demonstrated that being pushed can prompt gorging, expanded craving, voraciously consuming food and weight increase.

There are numerous straightforward approaches to diminish your regular feelings of anxiety. Think about utilizing yoga, tuning in to music, planting, reflection, exercise and breathing strategies.

Stress can prompt indulging, so diminishing the worry in your regular day to day existence is one significant advance you can take to stop this descending winding.

Try and Have Mindful Eating

Receiving careful eating systems is perhaps the most ideal approaches to avert indulging. The act of careful eating stresses the significance of concentrating on the present minute and monitoring your musings, feelings and faculties while devouring nourishment.

Numerous studies have demonstrated that careful eating is a successful method to decrease gorging practices, indulging and passionate eating.

Eating all the more gradually, taking little chomps, biting completely, monitoring your faculties and valuing your nourishment are largely basic care rehearses you can join into your every day schedule.

The act of careful eating has been appeared to help diminish voraciously consuming food practices. Careful eating centers around monitoring your musings and faculties while eating.

Skipping dinners may make you overeat later in the day — instead, center around keeping yourself feeling fulfilled by eating offset suppers made with entire nourishments.

Keep a Food Journal

Monitoring what you eat in a nourishment journal or versatile application may help diminish indulging.

Numerous studies have indicated that utilizing self-observing procedures like keeping a nourishment journal may help with weight reduction.

Furthermore, utilizing a nourishment diary can make you increasingly mindful of circumstances where you are destined to overeat and food sources that you will, in general, binge on.

Studies have indicated that following your nourishment admission may assist you with shedding pounds. It will likewise assist you with getting increasingly mindful of your propensities.

Eat With Like-Minded Friends

The nourishment decisions of your feasting sidekicks may have more effect on your nourishment consumption than you understand.

Various ponders have discovered that individuals' nourishment decisions are vigorously affected by the individuals they eat with.

You may, in general, eat comparative sums as people around you, so eating out with companions who indulge may make you overeat too.

Also, contemplates have demonstrated that an individual is increasingly disposed to arrange undesirable alternatives if their eating accomplice does.

Deciding to eat with loved ones who have comparative wellbeing objectives can assist you with remaining on course and decrease your odds of indulging.

Who you eat with may significantly affect your nourishment decisions. Attempt to eat with individuals who additionally need to eat hearty suppers in moderate segments.

Top off on Protein

Protein helps keep you full for the day and can diminish the craving to indulge.

For instance, having a high-protein breakfast has been appeared to decrease hunger and eating later in the day.

Picking a protein-rich breakfast like eggs will, in general, lower levels of ghrelin, a hormone that invigorates hunger.

Including higher-protein snacks, for example, Greek yogurt to your routine can likewise assist you with eating less for the day and monitor hunger.

Eating protein-rich nourishments may assist you with fighting off appetite and yearnings. Beginning the day with a high-protein breakfast can likewise help battle with craving later in the day.

Balance out Your Blood Sugar Levels

Eating white bread treats, sweets and different starches with high glycemic records will probably cause your glucose levels to spike, at that point, fall rapidly.

This fast glucose variance has been appeared to advance craving and can prompt indulging.

Picking nourishments with lower glycemic files will help avoid glucose spikes and may diminish indulging. Beans, oats, and dark colored rice are, for the most part, incredible alternatives.

Eat nourishments that help keep your glucose levels steady. High-glycemic nourishments like treats and white bread can make your glucose spike at that point drop, which may prompt indulging. Instead, pick nourishments like beans, oats and dark colored rice.

Slow Down

Rapid eating may make you indulge and can prompt weight increase after some time.

Slow-paced eating is related to expanded completion and diminished hunger and can fill in as a valuable device for controlling overeating.

Setting aside the effort to altogether bite nourishment has likewise been appeared to decrease generally nourishment admission and increment sentiments of completion.

Concentrating on eating all the more gradually and biting your nourishment completely may assist you with perceiving indications of totality and may decrease uncontrollable eating.

Watch Your Alcohol Intake

Drinking liquor may make you indulge by bringing down your restraints and invigorating your hunger.

While having a beverage or two with a feast won't have an immense impact, having a few drinks in a single sitting may prompt expanded degrees of appetite.

One study found that understudies who drank four to five drinks one after another more than once seven days were bound to gorge after drinking contrasted with understudies who drank each to two drinks in turn.

Reducing the measure of liquor you drink might be a decent method to limit excessive eating.

Studies show that drinking a few beverages in a single sitting may lead you to bingeee. Instead, stick to only a couple of beverages, or do without drinking liquor altogether.

Plan Ahead

In case you're not readied when the craving strikes, you're bound to settle on poor nourishment decisions that can lead you to overeat.

In case you're compelled to buy dinners and snacks, finally, from cafés or shops, you're bound to settle on unpopular decisions and eat more than you should.

Instead, keep sound tidbits close by, pack home-prepared snacks, and stock your ice chest with reliable alternatives so you can get ready supper at home.

These systems will assist you in reducing indulging. Also, making more suppers at home can set aside your cash and time.

The more you set up a plan to eat heartily, the more outlandish you are to overeat. Keep your cooler and wash room loaded with solid, filling nourishments.

Replace Sugary Beverages With Water

Drinking sugary refreshments like pop and squeeze could prompt weight pick up and build your danger of specific sicknesses like diabetes.

Studies have demonstrated that devouring improved beverages with dinners might be connected to indulging also.

An audit of 17 considers found that grown-ups who drank sugar-improved drinks with dinners devoured 7.8% more nourishment than adults who expended water with suppers.

Picking water or unsweetened seltzer over improved refreshments may help lessen overeating.

Keep away from sugary refreshments. They are linked with the risk of diabetes and different infections, and may likewise be connected to indulging. Drink water.

Check in With Yourself

Do you end up going to the kitchen and checking the refrigerator excessively regularly?

If you overeat when you are not eager, it might be a smart thought to pause for a while to comprehend why you incline to eat.

Despondency and weariness are two typical issues that have been connected to the desire to eat uncontrollably.

Luckily, there are some steps to take if you need to break the cycle. For instance, try another movement you appreciate. It might help counteract weariness and occupy you from the inclination to snack.

If you accept wretchedness might be driving your excessive feeding, search out psychological wellness experts for direction. They can assist you with refocusing.

Wonder why you're indulging and address the issues behind the conduct. Sorrow and fatigue are two typical reasons. If you believe you're encountering wretchedness, search out emotional well-being proficient for direction.

Discard the Diet Mentality

Prevailing fashion eats fewer carbs presumably won't assist you with halting indulging over the long haul. Present moment, restrictive diets may prompt fast weight reduction; however, they are frequently unsustainable and can set you up for disappointment.

Instead, make long haul way of life changes that advance wellbeing and health. It's the ideal approach to make a reasonable association with nourishment and avert propensities like gorging.

Rather than going on prevailing fashion diets to control your indulging, locate a reasonable method for eating that supports your body and causes you to arrive at ideal wellbeing.

Bring an end to Old Habits

Habits can be challenging to break, particularly when they include nourishment.

Numerous individuals get into agreeable schedules, such as having supper before the TV or having a bowl of frozen yogurt consistently.

It might require some investment to distinguish unfortunate practices that lead you to indulge and supplant them with new, solid propensities; however, it's certainly justified regardless of the exertion.

For instance, make it a point to have during supper rather than before the TV, or replace your daily bowl of frozen yogurt with a hot cup of tea. These substitutions will become solid habits after some time.

Recognize your unfortunate propensities, and step by step, supplant them with new, progressively positive practices.

Eat Healthy Fats

Albeit high-fat nourishments are frequently connected with weight addition and indulging, picking nourishments wealthy in sound fats can assist you with eating less.

A few reports have indicated that grown-ups who devour high-fat, low-carb abstains from food are less eager three to four hours after suppers and lose more weight after some time than individuals who expend slims down high in carbs and low in fat.

Including sound fats like avocados, nuts, seeds, nut spreads, and olive oil to your eating regimen may assist you with feeling progressively fulfilled after suppers and lessen indulging.

Have a go at adding progressively healthy fats to your eating routine. Studies have demonstrated it might assist you with feeling satisfied after suppers and get thinner over the long haul.

Remember Your Goals

Setting short-and long haul objectives and alluding to them regularly may assist you with remaining on following and lessen the inclination to indulge.

Knowing why you need to quit gorging and how indulging is shielding you from arriving at your wellbeing and health objectives can persuade you to bring an end to this undesirable propensity.

Writing down persuasive statements and placing them in prominent places around your home can help you with the right inspiration to adhere to your arrangement.

Recognize explicit short-and long haul eating objectives and allude to them frequently. It can even be useful to put inspirational statements around your home.

Find support If You Need It

BED, which we have discussed earlier, is a genuine dietary problem described by manifestations that incorporate over and over gorging on massive amounts of nourishment, a feeling of loss of control during eating, and sentiments of blame or pain after a gorge.

BED influences a great many individuals worldwide and is the most well-known dietary issue in the United States.

If you feel that you may have Binge Eating Disorder, it's critical to find support. Talk with your primary care physician or another certified wellbeing proficient about treatment choices.

If you usually binge on vast amounts of nourishment, feel lost control, and sentiments of blame, you should look for expert assistance.

Practical Steps to Take

Make an 80/20 Scheme

There is nothing like a perfect human. Similarly, no one will observe any specific diet scheme perfectly. In reality, indulging in some of the "fun" food items that your plan might classify as off limits are sometimes beneficial. Some diet schemes are not flexible to follow as they cut off too many foods. If a food item is completely banned in your scheme, focusing on it will be too easy. One of the risks that this brings is that you get too concerned with those "prohibited" foods that intensify the desire and stress to consume them. Occasionally it's good to have "fun;" in fact, some food schemes even call for a cheat day.

The truth is that now and then consuming an extra ice cream chocolate bar or scoop will not destabilise your scheme. And that is why you need to use the 80–20 rule in your scheme. When 80 percent of what you eat on the schedule is nutritious, and the last 20 percent is off the schedule, you will still be effective at weight loss.

Nonetheless, some schemes don't want to encourage cheating because the people involved don't know when to quit. One cheat can result in an even greater cheat, and then you will be off the scheme.

You must learn to discipline yourself if you want to use a feeding scheme successfully. This approach isn't for you if you are the kind of person that gets a taste of candy or Milkshakes and can't stop eating or taking the whole item. It would be wise to follow the scheme as carefully as you can to steer clear of those cravings that make you go on a binge.

Make a Trigger List

Cravings from your surroundings will not suddenly vanish. Because these cravings are a prominent part of the world in which we live, having a strategy to deal with it is wise. This temptation program must be compact, readily available, and relatively straightforward to initiate in seconds.

My college baseball coach would consider it the principle of the five P's: "Proper Preparation Prevents Poor Performance." If you're ready for the likelihood of temptation, then you're going to perform well when it's necessary to fight anything that's attempting to get you in. Creating a plan is as simple as including more details of your trigger list.

Draw out a list, and create a three column table that includes a response that you need to choose, rather than giving in to the enticing food. If you have fresh ideas on how to escape from our cravings, attach them to the list. Create many copies and keep them in a strategic location where you can easily reach for a copy and use it, whether you're at home, working, or doing daily chores.

Example of a Trigger List

Cravings	Triggers	Alternative Response
Chocolate	Depressed/Paranoid	Call a friend and address the issue
Creamed Popcorn	Watching Movies	Eat Organic Snacks instead
Ice Cream	Criticisms/Rage	Jog or Write a Diary
French Fries	When in a traffic	Listen to favorite music or radio
Doughnuts	Hungry when in a rush	Keep some fruits in the car or office
Creamy Pasta	Tired and exhausted	Listen to music or meditate
Soda	When you are thirsty	Drink caffeinated tea without sugar

Resisting Temptations in Parties

We understand that throughout work lunches, dinner parties, or banquets, it can be enticing to deviate from your food scheme. Keep up the good fight and remain strong! Every moment you find yourself stuck in such situations that need some extra discipline, try the following helpful hints:

Carry Your Dish: one easy way to be self-disciplined at a business lunch or picnic food offerings is to carry your meal. Choose a vegetarian option that fits for you and your schedule, and it will be an excellent option for other customers who are also conscious of their weight loss goals.

Keep a Bottle of Water with you: Keep in your right hand a bottle of water. Since you already carry a bottle of water, it will become harder for you to grab any accessible food quickly. You can take a refreshing gulp of hydrating water rather than picking up baked goods that are detrimental to your health. That is a win-win approach.

Eat before the party starts: If you are filled at the beginning of the party, you would not want to binge on snacks. Previously eating will keep you feeling strong when you're enticed with party snacks!

Chew Gum: In case you don't know, most of these helpful hints are centered around keeping your mind away from the urge to binge. Chewing sugar-free gum is a great way to do just that. This keeps your mouth busy and serves as an additional craving barrier!

Don't give up: be sure to pardon yourself if you got side-tracked your schedule. One moment of lack of self-control will NOT deny all of your past achievements. Cherish your success and keep it going! It will get better.

Conclusion

Numerous individuals battle with emotional eating.

Luckily, there are numerous approaches to assume back responsibility for your dietary patterns.

For instance, have a go at adding more protein to your suppers, actualizing careful eating methods, and lessening your feelings of anxiety.

Social insurance experts like clinicians, specialists, or enlisted dietitians can likewise give advising and direction to assist you with refocusing.

Overeating can be a hard habit to overcome. However, you can do it. Utilize these tips to assist yourself with building up another fixed daily schedule, and make a point to look for expert assistance if you need it.

Chapter Six: Diet Management Basics

In nutritional science, diet is commonly used to refer to the amount of food consumed by a person. More often than not, it is construed in the context of a weight management plan. That is a laid-out plan containing specific consumption of nutrients for weight loss. Also, people might have preferences in terms of choosing foods to consume. This may be due to culture or individual perception of the food. In essence, people make their diet, and it is of two ways – either it is balanced and healthy or not.

It should be noted that a balanced nutrition plan requires the consumption of most, if not all, the six classes of nutrients, namely; Carbohydrates, Protein, Water, Lipids, Minerals, and Vitamins. All these are needed for the body to function and maintain great shape. A typical diet should have about 55% Carbohydrates, 5% Protein, and Fats not exceeding 30%.

The choice of food we consume and our nutritional habits have significant roles to play in our lives as they affect our lives and the quality of life we live, our health, and on the long run, our longevity. Health professionals may advise a reduction in the intake of certain foods for health reasons, which might slightly not follow the nutritional order. But in general cases, it is essential to create a diet plan that contains all the vital nutrients necessary for the body to thrive.

The benefits of consuming the right foods in the right amount or following the right consumption plan cannot be overemphasized. Apart from the biological functions that foods offer, they also have emotional importance. We would take a closer look at all that a healthy diet plan has to offer now.

Benefits of A Good Diet Plan

If you were told that you could control your mood, increasing your mental abilities, and overall productivity by doing just one thing – eating, would you take it? I know I would, and without giving it a second thought. In the literal sense of it, it is considered that we are what we eat. That means we can also dictate what we eat in order to achieve the goals we have for our bodies.

The benefits of eating healthily (the activation of a healthy or balanced diet plan) would be structured in two forms, which are the biological benefits and emotional benefits. The emotional benefits, as we will see, does not imply that we have to eat emotionally.

I should restate emphatically that emotional eating is not as ideal as it neither solves the problem nor gives lasting comfort. Instead, it could birth another set of negative emotions. On the other hand, however, healthy eating does not mean you eat to correct or manage your feelings either. The emotional importance would be considered to give a deeper knowledge.

Biological Benefits

The benefits here are the most commonly talked about and usually easily identifiable. This is because they somehow involve the stomach and our physiological health. As we will see, a healthy balanced diet does a lot to our body system.

- Weight Management

If you ask anybody why they create a diet plan, more often than not, the answer would be to control weight. It is true. One of the most effective ways to control your weight is by creating a diet plan that works for that purpose.

Most people use diet plans to reduce weight. Losing weight reduces the risk of severe health issues because people with abnormal weight have the tendency of developing issues such as heart disease, some cancers, and reduced bone solidity.

- Defense Wall And A Fight Against Diseases

A diet plan prevents the outbreak of diseases. Food perfects our health. Creating a healthy eating plan will allow us to only focus on foods that contain nutrients that our bodies need to defend against diseases. Examples are vegetables, eggs, apples, alfalfa sprouts, and avocados.

- Energy

Under-eating is a bad habit, but overdoing it is not so good either. A diet plan helps you regulate how much you eat while you still get to enjoy the physical energy boost food offers.

- Good And Healthy Sleep

Diet plan helps control eating habits that tend to disrupt our sleep. When you create a diet plan, you are able to decide which food to consume and the quantity of the food.

- Longevity

This is not a magic trick, but it does work like one. When you stick to your diet plan, you increase your chance of a long life. The combination of fruits, vegetables, together with timely exercise, would go a long way in deciding how long you will live.

Other biological benefits of a diet plan include:

- It gives strong bones and teeth.

- Improves heart health and prevents stroke.

- Gives clearer and finer skin.

- Overall growth and physical development.

- Saves money.

Psychological Or Emotional Benefits

A healthy diet has an important role to play in our mental health. What we eat affects how our immune systems operate, how our genes work, and how our bodies respond. It should nonetheless be noted that eating does not and should not be made as a substitute for medication and other mental treatments. Below are the emotional benefits of a healthy diet plan.

- Mood Enhancement

Various studies have shown that there is a relationship between the food we eat and our moods. Although there are also indications that the effects of foods on moods vary depending on the individual. But, the general advice is that people should consume foods which are rich in proteins, contain low fats, and a reasonable amount of carbohydrates. The presence of these three generally improves the moods of most people.

- Brain Functions

Eating a balanced meal rich in nutrients boosts the brain's functions. How much your brain can do depends on how healthy you eat. Therefore, if you want a healthier brain, you have to eat healthier. Nutritionists recommend that you eat foods like freshly brewed tea, wild salmon, blueberries, and a reasonable amount of chocolate.

- Emotional Energy Levels

When we undertake a healthy diet plan, we would always enjoy the rush of energy and experience a higher level of productivity. Experts recommend the consumption of food that contains carbs, fats, vegetables, proteins as well as whole grains.

You can get a quick energy boost when you concentrate on healthy snacks like fruits, nuts and low fat yoghurts.

You also need to concentrate on take adequate quantity of water and limit caffeine and sugar to the barest minimum. Doing this will help keep your energy level in check by regulating it.

- No Depression

Eating foods that contain a balanced composition of nutrients reduces the risk of mental health problems like depression. To keep your mind in a sharp state and active, you need nutrients like vitamins and minerals. Research has shown that the deficiency of the B12 vitamins, calcium, and iron in the body usually contributes to anxiety and depression.

A study was conducted by researchers at the National Institute of Health. The study revealed that a close examination of the food intake habit of depressed people reveals that they are lacking in many essential diets. In other words, they might even be guilty of eating foods that will feed their depression

They recommend minerals like zinc, selenium, amino and fatty acids, and magnesium. Drinking a lot of water is also an excellent way to stay active. However, eating does not solve the problem of depression or anxiety; it can only prevent possible occurrence.

- Ability To Learn

"Healthy diet is primal to learning, it improves social behaviors and could also help people develop interactive skills." says Dr. JoQueta Handy. A good and healthy diet keeps your brain in the smart mode, ensuring healthy brain activity. Breakfast is crucial, though. Starting the day with nutrient-filled breakfast improves your cognitive performance.

Diet Management

The term diet management can also be referred to as food management. It simply means the process of handling and providing the best nutritional options for diet planning. It involves the careful formation of diet plans that work for individuals. Certain factors are to be considered in doing this. They include personal preference, food availability, financial capacity, and tradition. It is possible to create a perfect diet plan by putting in all these factors.

Diet management can be done individually, and you can also seek the help of a nutritionist. But it is more effective if you do this by yourself. All you need is your heart, commitment, focus, pen, and a piece of paper.

Creating A Diet Plan

Creating your own personalized diet plan is the first step to managing your diet. Or would you work on another person's food plan? We all have different diet goals, so it is advisable to create your diet plan by yourself, especially if you are just starting out.

People are often aware of their health and understand the importance of making healthy food selections. But they do not know how to organize their foods or find it challenging doing so. Here, steps or tips, as you may call them, on how to create your own personalized diet plan will be given.

How To Create Your Diet Plan

The following are simple steps you can take in creating your diet plan.

- List out your health goals.
- Calculate and be aware of your calorie intake.
- Know the nutrients in every meal.
- Know and understand the portion sizes of the different food groups.

- Go for healthy organic foods rather than processed and junk foods. For instance, choose vegetables, whole grains, and fruits.

- Be versatile in your schedule. Mix meals up. You do not have to eat the same set of meals every day.

- Know your mealtimes. Or choose the number of times you want to eat each day, which is usually three or four times. This would help you know how to fix the perfect mix every day.

- Write your schedule.

- Choose a method to input your schedule. You can employ Word, Excel, or other specific food schedule and tracking apps. Using apps is much easier because when you fill in your meal plan for each day, you would be able to calculate the number of macronutrients and calories you take. This is notably better as it saves time.

Maintaining A Daily Journal

There is no better way to track your food consumption that recording it in a journal. A study has shown that keeping a food journal aids weight loss program, and those who keep a food journal tend to lose twice as much weight as people who do not.

A food journal is a recording tool to check in with your food consumption. Also, it is used to record how you feel before, during, and after you eat. A published result of a study in Obesity has shown that it takes less than fifteen minutes a day to track what you eat every day. Therefore, since it does not take time, monitoring food consumption using a journal should be what every dieter should do.

How To

Pen and paper is a reliable way to do it. But if it cannot work effectively for you, try using your phone notepad or an app.

- Write down the food the very moment you are eating them.
- Note down where and what you are doing while eating.
- Record the feelings you experience while you eat.
- Do not forget what you have missed. This may be skipping a meal or eating what your colleague at work brought for you. It can also be some toppings that came with your order, record everything.
- To thy own self be true. It is a food journal – only you can see it. You do not have to lie and put your health at risk.
- Stay positive. If what you record at the end of the day does not match your expectations, do not worry. The whole essence of keeping a food journal is to monitor what and how much you take. It will help you make the necessary adjustments to your diet plan.

Benefits Of Maintaining A Food Journal

Why do you want to keep a food journal? Whether your reason is to become healthier or because you want to lose weight, keeping a food journal can help make whatever change you desire. Below is a list of proved benefits keeping a food journal has to offer.

- Food journal aids weight loss.
- Rerecording your reaction before, during, and after meals helps you determine your food intolerances.

- It keeps you aware of the portions of food you consume, and you are able to control them.

- It records nutrition facts. This way, you are able to determine what nutrients you are not having enough and what food you reduce its intake.

- It can help identify triggers of emotional and unhealthy eating.

Stick To Your Healthy Diet Plan

- Have Realistic Goals

Everyone wants a perfect weight. So it is easy to set a diet plan for that purpose. However, did you know that the feasibility of achieving your diet plan goals is dependent on the expectations you set for yourself? Let us assume you want to lose weight, for instance. If you throw yourself into unnecessary pressure by setting up a diet plan that keeps you inconvenient, you might end up not reaching that target.

In essence, it is better to have realistic expectations. Doing this increases the chances of success, and it would keep you motivated to set higher goals. Start from the small ones.

- Rid yourself of unhealthy foods or foods outside your diet plan

Have you heard of the statement, "out of sight, out of mind"? It means what you do not see; you do not consider it. If you keep foods that are outside your diet plan in your kitchen or any other place you can easily access, the diet plan would not work. This is because you would always want to have a taste, and it cannot help you in achieving your diet goals.

- Get Into Mindful Eating

Practicing mindful eating is an excellent way to maintain your diet. Being mindful involves the conscious recognition of the foods you eat as necessary consumptions that your body needs. It is like appreciating the food for the nourishing value it provides. Mindful eating also requires that you are conscious and intentional about the amount of food you consume. This is to make sure that you do not eat out of order and fall into binge eating.

- Remember What Motivates You

Nobody makes a diet plan out of the blue moon. They have their reasons for doing so. Your diet plan is expected to indicate your current state and where you intend to be by the time you progress with the plan. So, while it is not easy to stick with the plan, you can regularly remind yourself why you are doing it in the first place and what you hope to achieve at the end of the day.

- Do not forget the healthy snacks

Sometimes, we might be away from home for an extended period, and it is rather tough, if not impossible, to continue with our diet plans. During times such as this, when we become hungry, we might be tempted to pick anything the mouth can eat, which might not be helpful to us. By grabbing whatever is available, we become vulnerable to eating processed foods that do not really quench our hunger nor do any good to our bodies on the long run.

One way to still ensure that you are on the right track on your diet plan is carrying healthy snacks with you as you travel. Snacks high in protein come in handy in this instance. This way, you can control your appetite until you can have a full meal. Examples of high-protein foods include peanuts, jerky, cheese, and almonds.

- Plan before eating out

If you have to go out with your colleagues after work hours, it is best to have a plan. It is usually challenging to stick to your diet plan if you are not eating in your home. But if you find yourself in a restaurant, check out what is on the menu before you order. In case you find nothing you would like, consider drinking only water, especially if you are not hungry.

- Deal With Workplace Junks

You might be given a break in your workplace and have the chance to grab a few bites from the food joint near your office. In some companies, there is usually a small part of the buildings designed to house snacks and drinks for their workers. Careful not to fall for snacks that do not fulfill your diet plan.

To make it easy for you, plan your day before leaving in the morning. Package foods that do not spoil quickly and challenge yourself to stick to your plan no matter the charm of the snacks on the table.

- Do Not Skip Breakfast

Working-class people who need to get to work as early as possible tend to skip breakfast. The result is that they get hungry immediately. They start work, and the urge to keep going might become unbearable. As a result, they are ready to die for anything they could find and eat. Getting hungry later might lead to binge eating. In other words, never skip breakfast. You can make time for morning meals like cereal high in fiber, fruits, and low-fat milk.

- Sleeping And Meditation

When you deprive yourself of sleep, your body produces in excess, ghrelin, a hormone that stimulates the appetite. So when you do not sleep when your body needs it, you would always want to be eating.

Meditation also helps sharpen your mind to concentrate on your diet and feel contented with what you eat. Sleeping and meditating would make you feel rested while also preventing you from unnecessary eating.

- Beware Of Nighttime Snacks

One of the easiest ways to fall off course from your diet plan is by encouraging yourself to snack after dinner. That is when mindless eating mostly occurs. Some people cannot watch TV without snacking. If you are like that, practice closing the kitchen after dinner or opt for snacks with low calories.

- Stay Hydrated

Never run short on water. Drink plenty of it or other beverages that do not contain calories. Sometimes, we confuse thirst with hunger and end up eating to the point of discomfort when an ice-cold bottle of water is all we need. When next you feel you are hungry, try drinking water before eating, you might be surprised that your supposedly hungry stomach is satisfied. If water does not go, consider a bottle of flavored water or a cup of herbal tea containing fruit.

- Monitor Your Progress

You can quickly ditch your diet plan if you do not monitor how far you have gone. Keeping tabs on your performance would let you how well you have done and how productive the plan has been. As you record your work and progress levels, you can discover where you need to make an adjustment. This would help focus on increasing your performance and ensure that you are moving in the right direction to achieve your diet goals.

Other useful tips on how to keep your diet plan intact

- Have protein during every meal.
- Break your calories into smaller snacks during the day.
- Have fiber in your diet.
- Limit alcohol intake.
- Eat fruits and vegetables.
- Do not give up.

Chapter Seven: How Exercise And Meditation Can Help Reduce Triggers

Emotional eating is not something you should joke with. If you consider the implications, you would understand that it goes beyond hiding behind your emotions by eating – and eventually overeating. The complications include both psychological and physiological effects. To keep out of emotional eating; therefore, one must exercise a conscious effort to deal with what might turn a frequent occurrence.

There are a number of possible ways to correct emotional eating. But instead of fighting the very act itself, why not practice control over the triggers. That is, get over the triggers, so you do not have to struggle with the habit. This conception is couched in the famous statement that "prevention is better than cure." It is easier to overcome emotional eating if you treat the triggers.

According to findings, there are two very effective ways to control the triggers that birth emotional eating. These are Exercise and Meditation. It should be noted that these two ways have existed for long, tested, and confirmed as potent ways to deal with emotional eating triggers, thereby preventing the occurrence of emotional eating itself.

This chapter will give exhaustive explanations on Exercise and Meditation, how they help reduce emotional eating triggers, and easy tips on how to go about doing them. In order to understand what this chapter will talk about, let us list what we will be dealing with, that is the triggers mentioned in chapter one of this book. The triggers include:

- Emotions.
- Habits.
- Fatigue.
- Boredom.
- External Influence.
- For Pleasure.

Exercise

Have you been advised to run a few miles every morning? Or hit the gym every evening? For good physical health, doctors might prescribe exercising the body. In reality, very few people consider exercise as having mental benefits. They usually associate exercise with weight loss, increase in strength, and aerobic capacity. So, more often than not, they do not believe that exercise has anything to do with their mental health.

Exercise involves practicing physical activities to increase the heart rate beyond normal levels. It is an essential method of improving and preserving physical and mental health. It can come in different forms. Whether you opt for light exercises such as a short walk, or exercise with a high intensity such as uphill running or weightlifting, exercise generally provides considerable benefits to the mind and body.

In other words, exercise is any activity that involves body movements to enhance or improve the physiological composition of the body and maintain overall health. Exercise is undertaken for various reasons. It might be for medical reasons – usually directed by health physicians and nutritionists. It can also be for personal reasons to stay fit and in shape. For whatever reason or reasons you choose to exercise, you should know that it is an excellent way to preserve your health and develop a healthy lifestyle for yourself.

Everybody can relate to what exercise is and have few tips for keeping the body fit. Sadly, people would rather spend their time sitting at home or staying up late at work. Even when they eventually have some free time, they end up in front of the TV or with their phones. All these activities make us less active than we should.

This is so because we neglect to put our bodies to the physical test in order to improve it and maintain the general wellness of the body and mind. First, before we consider the importance of exercise, it is necessary to take a look at the statistics that have been recorded on exercise.

Statistics On Exercise

There are thousands of books on exercise that you could pick up and find millions of ideas on exercise. This is not to challenge their professionalism. The benefits of exercise cannot be overemphasized. As a result of the widely-spread recognition of exercise, many pieces of research on exercise have been conducted. And many are still going on at this present moment. So, let us dive straight into the facts and figures available on exercise.

- On a global scale, 81 percent of adolescents are not satisfactorily active.
- Exercise decreases the risk of heart disease by more than 20 percent.
- Every day, children spend more than 7 hours in front of the TV, computers or playing video games.
- Regular exercise lowers the risk of dementia by 30 percent.
- Exercise decreases the risk of diabetes by 50 percent.
- Exercise makes you smarter.
- According to WHO, the lack of exercise is one of the leading risk factors contributing to the global mortality rate.
- From a study, only one out of every three children is physically active every day.
- In the US, only 5 percent of adults undertake 30 minutes of physical activities each day.
- Only one out of every three adults participate and complete the recommended amount of physical activity each week.
- In 2006, a meta-analysis of 11 studies was conducted. The reports showed that depressed people who performed aerobic exercise improved equally as those given antidepressants.

Why Exercise

"I have a moderate weight, so why do I need to exercise?" "I want to, but what do I gain?"

How would you like to be active? And I mean super-active. Not the kind that you end up with weakened joints and pains all over your body after the day's work. How would you like to be still able to walk to the fridge, pick a bottle of cold water, and read the newspaper?

You already recognize that exercise is good, or at least you know a couple of people who look agile, fit, and seem to be always active. But do you know how good it is? It is a lot more than shedding fats or building muscles.

Consider a car that works every day. Sooner or later, it would begin to develop problems unless it is checked, maintained, and improved. It is the same with our bodies. We need constant maintenance and what better option could we choose than exercise. Below are what you stand to gain from regular exercise.

- Weight Management

Exercise keeps your body maintained, and if you desire to do without a few pounds, you can create an exercise plan for that purpose.

- Memory Improvement

Many studies indicated that exercise tends to boost memory and improve learning ability. This is because exercise surges the oxygen levels and blood flows in the brain. As a result, brain chemicals that produce cells in the hippocampus are released. The hippocampus is the area of the brain that controls learning and memory.

As a result of all these processes, cognitive ability, awareness, and concentration levels are boosted, thereby strengthening brain functions as well as reducing the risk of cognitive degenerative diseases such as Alzheimer's.

- Muscles And Bones

Exercise aids in the release of hormones that increase the ability of your muscles to absorb amino acids, which help their growth and prevent breakdown.

It also helps build strong bones and ensures that the tendons, joints, and ligaments are flexible. This would, in turn, enhance balance and coordination, reduce the risk of joint and back pains.

- Better Sleep

Exercise makes you tired. Essentially helping you to sleep healthily. A quality sleep activates a rest mode for your brain and body and helps reduce stress.

- Bad Day For Stress

We all have to experience stress, and it can wreak havoc in our lives if not treated. One way to manage stress is by exercising. When you exercise, your body release stress fighters called endorphins. Also, exercise helps clear your mind, thereby reducing stress.

Other benefits include:

- Exercise increases energy levels.
- It makes you happier.
- It decreases the risk of chronic diseases.
- It gives a better posture.
- Long life.

Doing It

If you really want to start, then you need to know what you are doing. Exercise falls into four main categories, and briefly, we will discuss them.

- Aerobic

It is the most common perception of exercise. It involves training to build fitness levels. This exercise makes you breathe harder and speeds up the heart rate. Aerobic exercise lowers blood pressure, boosts mood, burn fats, aids weight loss program, among others.

You can perform this exercise by running, cycling, dancing, or any other physical activity that requires movement.

- Balance Exercise

This includes activities that aid balance by building your core strength. It is mostly undertaken by people who cannot hold themselves together and tend to fall. Examples of this exercise are yoga and tai chi.

- Strength Development

Bodyweight activities like push-ups and squats will do the job and provide strength for your muscles.

In fact, your body is one of the best accessories to help with your workout activities.

* Flexibility

Stretching is the best guess here. It is essential, but it is often overlooked when talking about exercise. Flexibility improves your quality of life. Imagine not being able to bend correctly to pick a toy for a kid or struggling with reversing your car because you could not look over your shoulder.

Stretching reduces the risk of muscle cramps, strains, joint pain, and muscle damage.

Meditation

Meditation is a potent method used to train the mind. Meditation is a skillful practice that involves emerging with a new sense of awareness and getting a healthy sense of perception. It is a means of observing your feelings without necessarily turning them off. Instead, you perceive them in a dimension that gives you a sense of peace, freedom, and control.

Meditation is simple and can be practiced by anyone It takes patience and concentration, which you may have to struggle with at first.

Meditation is an act and comprises any or a set of techniques used in order to create a heightened state of mindfulness and focused attention. Spiritual leaders, educators, and mental health experts have developed tons of techniques that could be used in Meditation. These techniques are so much that everyone would find at least one that works for him. The idea is that although Meditation creates the chance to improve the mental and physical wellbeing, there is no totally right way to meditate. Therefore, people can choose whichever technique goes well with their personality, religion, lifestyle, or personal interest.

Few Things About Meditation

- Almost all religions such as Christianity, Islam, Buddhism, and Judaism, have their ways and methods of practicing Meditation.
- Meditation has roots in almost all cultures all over the world and could be traced back to thousands of years.
- Meditation can be used as religious practices as wells as for individual purposes.
- Meditation can also be a therapeutic technique.

Statistics On Meditation

Due to the benefits that are being attributed to Meditation, it has continued to gain a skyrocketing recognition. People are embracing Meditation, and the numbers keep increasing. No surprise there, Meditation is really doing a lot. Let us consider some statistics recording the Meditation trend.

- Meditation reduces anxiety by 60 percent.
- Meditation increases productivity by 120 percent.

- An estimated number of 500 million people meditate worldwide. The numbers keep increasing.
- 30 percent of those suffering from back pain experience improvement as they meditate compared to those using medication.
- Meditation reduces insomnia by 50 percent.
- Meditation reduces depression by 12 percent.
- Mindfulness Meditation reduces symptoms of Post-traumatic Stress Disorder (PTSD) by 73 percent.
- Meditation lowers blood pressure by 80 percent.

Benefits Of Meditation

The recognition of Meditation is increasing. This is due to the benefits that people are deriving from it. Although why people meditate could be attributed to individual reasons, nonetheless, there are scientifically proved health benefits of Meditation. Some of them include:

- Meditation reduces stress.
- Keeps anxiety at bay.
- Enhances self-awareness.
- Increases concentration or focus level.
- Prevents memory loss and improves cognitive ability.
- Defends against addictions.
- Develops a positive mindset.
- Helps control negative emotions — for example, pain, sadness, and disappointment.
- Reduces the risk of high blood pressure.
- Betters sleep.

How To Meditate

One thing you must note is that the purpose of Meditation is to create mindfulness and to make all your negative emotions and thoughts disappear magically. So, practicing Meditation for you should be about breathing to keep your mind calm, at peace, and in control.

Meditation could be simple as well as hard, depends on the way you perceive it. However, it gets hard when you begin to struggle with keeping your concentration. In any way, Meditation is what everyone must practice, especially if you are the type that has too much going on. Below is a list of tips to get you started into meditation.

- Find a comfortable place.
- Sit and sit still for a few minutes. Make sure you are comfortable.
- Set a time limit for your practice.
- Concentrate on your breath. Feel and follow as it goes and comes.
- Be aware when your mind has wandered. Do not worry, this happens.
- Do not be mad about your wandering mind. Gently recover your concentration.
- Stay on it.
- Round up gently. Gently open your eyes and feel your body.

To stay in the right mind, you need Meditation. And it is essential to make it a habit. One way to ensure you practice it on a regular basis is by using a reminder. Clearing the mind ensures you are not vulnerable to unhealthy eating habits.

Exercise And Meditation Versus The Triggers

Throughout the explanations given on both exercise and Meditation, have you discovered how they help fight the triggers? To make your discovery easier, consider this analysis:

1.   All the triggers of emotional eating listed in this book, and some others go straight to and affect your mind/brain and not your body.

2.   Emotional eating is then activated in your mind/brain as a result of the triggers. That is, thinking about the emotions is creating an uncontrollable urge to eat.

3.   Exercise and Meditation are potent ways of ridding your mind of clutters, which in this case, includes the triggers. Exercise and Meditation renew your mind, increase awareness and concentration levels, and give you control over your mind.

Does the illustration work for you?

The first thing you must do is to identify the triggers. The first step to solving a problem is to know the source of the problem. So if you quickly want to quit emotional eating, you must identify the triggers. When you know what you are up against, employ these two methods (exercise and Meditation). Follow the steps listed to practice each of them and stick to it.

This is not to say it would be easy on the way, no, it is not. You need to exercise focus and commitment. If you fail at one point, get back up. You should focus on your targets and not the temporary pain of running every day or sitting in a position for a few minutes.

Also, the mind receives thousands of information and processes a lot of thoughts every day, so it does not have any automatic filter. That means you always need to filter it, remove the clutters like emotional eating triggers, and free your mind. This can be effectively done by regular exercise and Meditation. Remember, your mind is your warehouse. You must be conscious of what goes into it.

Chapter Eight: The Seven-Day Plan

Emotional eating is dangerous, risky, and can be life-sucking as it develops. Anybody can fall victim to emotional eating. To state the reality even, everyone you have met or will ever meet has done it sometimes in their lives. The frequent occurrence of emotional eating makes the matter worse. Some people are knee-deep in the act that they consider emotional eating part of their lives. They stop struggling with it and accept the condition as permanent. Sadly, it does not help them or the situations they face. Instead, it becomes much more difficult for them to live as pleased. They still have to struggle with the trigger-situations, the emotional reactions which have no expiry date while been consumed in the implications of emotional eating.

What people call a healthy desire for food might be the only problem that can redirect their lives and make them struggle to live a free, peaceful, and enjoyable lifestyle. Emotional eating goes beyond the stomach. It includes the brain, the mind, and all other essences of existence. Doing it is like relinquishing the control of your life. This is because while you emotionally eat to suppress or reward your emotions, you are developing the mentality which you can find sanctuary in food. Consequently, you are quick to run to food whenever anything out of expectation happens, causing you to rely on food even more than yourself.

Having explained all there is as regards emotional eating, including related terms, their complications, and various statistical analysis, it should, however, come as a relief that emotional eating can be done away with – for good. Unfortunately, there are some who suffer in the clamps of emotional eating in silence or fail to realize that they are emotional eaters, and they need help. As much as emotional eating is cancerous to the body and mind, the good news is that it can be removed. And it is even easy to overcome before it becomes a habit. Although, it should be noted that as long as emotional triggers are coming, the temptation to go back will always surface. So, while you are conscious of not overeating from emotions, you must also lookout for the triggers.

Overcoming emotional eating can be hard and easy at the same time. Of course, you do not suppose it is easy to recover power from what tends to control your mind. This chapter will deal with simple steps that can help you overcome the urge to overeating as a result of your emotions while also dealing with the triggers. These tips can be employed every day until you develop an unconscious control of emotional eating. But first, there is one essential thing that you must know before you start the journey of overcoming emotional eating.

Be Mindfully Prepared

Your mind is capable of many things, but this depends on what you do and how you treat it. To reiterate, you cannot always control what goes in, but you can decide how you handle it. What you want your mind to do is what it will do. Stephen Richards said, "You are essentially who you create yourself to be, and all that occurs in your life is the result of your own making." What does this mean to you? Does the idea of mind control pop up in your head?

The urge or hunger as the case may be, that births emotional eating comes from the mind – a mentality triggered by emotional reactions as a result of circumstances around or physical experiences. If emotional eating can be switched on through the mind, it is logical to conclude that the mind can as well put it off. And this is the case. Your mind is also involved in the fight against emotional eating. All you need to learn is how to position it so that the tiny little bit of control you have left over it can be put to maximum use.

How Do You Become Mindfully Prepared?

This is simply activating the mind and knowing what is and what is not and accepting it. Accepting it is not to believe there is nothing that can be done or that you have embraced what you call fate. Instead, you have to admit to the reality and situation of things.

To be mindfully prepared is to acknowledge the following about your situation on emotional eating:

- That you feel the urge to eat every time. You are experiencing emotional reactions and cannot seem to be able to control it.
- That you have developed the act of eating because of your emotions.
- That this act is already a habit or about to be.
- That there are complications and you have a victim of them.

- More importantly, having recognized the above, that you are ready to make conscious efforts to release yourself from the claws of emotional eating.

- Lastly, that it is possible to be free, and you are on that path to total control over emotional eating and the triggers.

In essence, for you to be able to control the emotional eating habit or perhaps remove it entirely from your life, you have to prepare your mind. When your mind is set in that motion, then whatever else you do is borne out of the mindset that "you have to fight it." And this is the right thing because the positive mindset will create in you the realization, commitment, and focus you need in achieving an emotional-eating-free life.

Having prepared your mind, we can start with a plan that will help you through the times of trying to set yourself free. Some might ask, "Why do I need my mind when I can just follow the plan?" or "why do I need a plan when I have my all-powerful mind?" well, the only answer I can give you is that you cannot do it without the two working together. Like an empire going for war, it needs the army general as well as the soldiers. The general directs the blood-thirsty soldiers, and they follow. In the same way, for you to win your war against emotional eating, you need your army general and your soldiers – your mind as the controller and your plans as the warriors.

The Seven-Day Plan

"I can stop emotional eating in seven days?"

It should be categorically stated that you would find tons of ways, plans, or steps to stop emotional eating on the internet. While some might actually work, some fail. This might be due to the complexities of some of the steps. In this chapter, however, there is a plan – a seven-day plan. This plan is expected to be carried out every day throughout the week, after which you start again. So, to answer the question above, while we cannot rule out the possibility of winning over emotional control after a week, we have to consider the kind of enemy we face here. This plan works, but it might take longer than a week – not very long, though, and you are sure to notice changes and development as you go on with it.

Lastly, as you work through the plan, you must have, on the other hand, try as much as possible to identify the emotional triggers. This is because recognizing the triggers would help you manage them and ultimately aid your efforts in overcoming emotional eating.

Now, here is the seven-day plan you should embark on to completely but gradually set yourself free from emotional eating.

- Plan Every Food And Snack
  The best way to stick to a healthy eating pattern is to make a conscious effort to arrange your order and quantity of food intake. Planning your breakfast, lunch, dinner, and snacks would help avoid mindless eating. Even if you should experience specific emotional reactions, you would be conscious of your eating schedule.

- Scanning And Checking

Another way to ensure that you eat intuitively is by scanning and checking your brain to discover what causes the hunger. In cases of emotional eating, hunger is usually triggered in the brain. So, if you do undertake this simple step every day, you would be able to decide which hunger is worth satisfying and which is not. Of course, you have to deal with emotional eating in another way other than eating.

- De-stress

This is a very powerful way to stay away from emotional eating. Emotional eating is easily triggered by stress. So make a conscious arrangement to stay away from stress. Not that it would not come to you, but that you have to keep it at bay. Exercise, positive affirmations, and meditation are useful techniques to de-stress.

- Never Stay Dehydrated

Most of the times, people confuse thirst for hunger. Add water to your daily plan. When you think you are hungry – rather unnecessarily, drink some water and see whether you would be okay or still remain hungry. Otherwise, you might end up overeating, thinking you are hungry when all your body needs a cold bottle of water.

- What Is On Your Mind

One of the ways to check if you are emotionally eating is to take notice of what is on your mind before you eat, while you eat, and after you are done eating. Record your actual observations and decide whether you are a victim of emotional eating or you are just fulfilling your body's need.

- Find The Triggers

This is somewhat easy. Emotional eating triggers create the urge to overeat to the point of physical discomfort uncontrollably. When this happens to you a couple of times, then you are emotionally eating.

Record the feelings or triggers, and devise means to have control over them.

- Stay Positive

Creating a positive mindset is the first step. But sticking to that sense of positivity is another task you must embrace if you want to overcome emotional eating. The trick to staying positive is to focus on what you want to do and what you must do. This, you should do instead of thinking about what you do not want to do.

- Know What Works For You

People who are over-confident in their abilities to handle emotional eating triggers are the ones who often end up in the pit. For instance, consider when you receive your salary at the end of the month that causes the joy you feel when going to the grocery store without a list. You might likely buy more than you need or consume a lot of snacks while you are shopping. In essence, know your strengths and weaknesses when it comes to eating habits. Try in every possible way not to do more than yourself and fall for your emotions. Instead, knowing and sticking to what works for you is an excellent way to stay in control.

- Snack Purposefully

Snack is good. Although over-consumption might lead to something else. However, plan your snack and eat it purposefully. There is a difference between snacking to help survive a stressful moment and eating snacks because you want to.

- Worry Less

Worry is a common occurrence, but you do not have to make it prompt you to overeat, because it can. Some people are fond of getting home from work, dropping their bags, and swiftly moving towards the kitchen to relief their feelings with the leftover cake or pizza. Instead of forming this habit, change your ritual, and enjoy other non-food activities such as switching on the TV, putting on music, or playing with your dog. Keep the worry outside the door!

• Declutter Your Home And Surrounding

A rough and untidy place has the tendency of creating emotions such as tiredness, laziness, and anxiety, which can be triggers of emotional eating. Get your home and surroundings clean and clear out the garbage.

• Always Improve Your Mood

You cannot be in a good mood all of the time. We would ever face challenges, circumstances, and outcomes that could alter our moods. When you experience a change in mood, you are likely to go into emotional eating as a result of trying to save yourself from the feelings. So instead of running to food as a cover, you can improve your mood by playing video games, taking a short walk, listening to music, and watching a sporting event.

• Exercise And Meditation

The benefits of these two cannot be overemphasized. They work wonders, and you would be surprised how fast you can recover and take control over emotional eating habit by doing these two. Exercise and meditation not only get us into good physical shape, but they also help clear our minds, activate a positive mindset, and grant us peace from within.

• Eat Healthy Foods

Eating healthy foods provides some form of satisfaction. In this way, you also prevent overeating. Satisfy your physical hunger with tasty and healthy foods, and you are sure to be able to keep your hands off overeating or unnecessary snacking.

Other tips you can add to the plan include:

- Find alternatives to food.

- Know when to stop eating.

- Talk to a friend.

- Focus on the positive changes and celebrate the little achievements.

The Healing Begins

These steps are not get-it-quick; hence, they cannot magically make your emotional eating habits disappear. It goes through processes that will readjust your mind. Also, it should be noted that practicing these steps every day does not automatically stop the urge to eat. In fact, it might likely intensify the urge at the beginning. So, while you have to avoid falling halfway into tempting cravings, you can also expect a gradual process of recovery and gaining of control. Eventually, you will get out of it and stay in charge of your emotional reactions and your eating habits.

Chapter Nine Learning the Joy of Eating Healthy

Deal with Food Obsessions

To benefit from your meals, you must discipline yourself against some food obsessions. Always pondering anything, including your nourishment, will overwhelm you and affect the way you eat. Nourishment is there to support your body and fulfill your spirit, but being obsessed with it is not proper.

Food obsessions are an aftereffect of individuals denying themselves of some food because of strict restrictions on their eating regimens and attempting to "control" their nourishment. In most cases, people do not even eat adequately, which could be an attempt to shed off some weight. However, this self-discipline can cause food obsessions.

How can you deal with food obsessions?

Pay attention to your body: Once you begin to pay close attention to your body and notice what it requires, eating well becomes less of a problem for you. Immediately start by observing how your body reacts after every meal. Are you exhausted, or are you feeling full of energy? Are you feeling nauseous or a little dizzy? Or are you very motivated and energized to take on the challenge? Be mindful of the interactions between what you eat and your body reactions afterward

Stay busy. Do everything you can to have a successful and complete day. It could appear oversimplified, but you can't be worried about what to eat every minute when you're preoccupied and engaged with so many workloads.

Shop and cook. Going shopping for food and preparing it by yourself — instead of getting supper at a neighborhood inexpensive restaurant or warming up a solidified supper — are proactive approaches to stop nourishment obsessions. In addition to the fact that they make you increasingly aware of your nourishment decisions, they will make you feel satisfied. This is because they help you to associate with what you're placing in your body. The straightforward demonstration of cooking your food likewise encourages you to set aside some effort to feed and accommodate your spirit.

Make an activity plan. An activity plan is a food timetable where you record what you will likely eat for the entire day. If you can work out a food timetable, working for the rest of the day would be easy as you tend to worry less about what to eat. Try not to stress if the arrangement doesn't turn out precisely; just the exercise alone is enough to reduce worry over food.

Accept who you are

There's a great deal of body shaming out there, and it's always about body size. While numerous men do not have any problems with how they look, this is by all accounts, an issue that mostly influences ladies. Be aware of this fact: Nobody has "a perfect body" because that term does not exist. The ideal body is something made and sustained by the media.

Being a woman means possessing curved hips, a rounded bottom, and broader thighs. Females have more waist circumference than males, and it is impossible to reverse that biological reality. The shapes and fats are how ladies have been made and grown; they need their rounded shapes to function effectively with their hormones, which will help them before, during, and after pregnancy.

Remember that, even if you spend most of your time working out, you can only become more lean and muscular. Still, you will never get the physique of famous people you see online. And, this has nothing to do with gender. Because of their genetic makeup, most models are quite lanky and lean; some eat, others don't. What they do to improve their body is solely based on their unique genes. It is not possible or practicable for everyone in the world to look like a model.

Stop Worrying over Scale Readings

Stop defining yourself with the number you see when you stand on scales. The main objective is to eat healthily and not to reach a number on a scale — which could be faulty. When you put all your attention on what a scale indicates, you risk being dominated by it.

Just like the world where you live, your body is always evolving, and every day you are going to weigh it again to find a different figure. For instance, if you decided to eat a salty meal yesterday night, your body can acquire five kilos of excess weight. Why will you disturb your peace with such fluctuations by what a system with automated digits tells you?

Merely choosing a "perfect" figure on your scale and then struggling to achieve it is not realistic for your body. Every figure you want will be meaningless because several factors will affect your ability to reach this number, most especially genetics. Alternatively, your perfect body should be defined by what should leave you feeling most proud of your body. It is the weight that leaves you feeling very healthy and lively.

Chapter 10: Learning to Move your body

Learning how to move your body effectively should be at the forefront of all you do in practice. Moving your body well is a form of taking full control of the way you display the energy of your body. It helps us to execute a challenging job and show gestures in a completely easy way.

If you can move your body well, you will easily find your inner power and strength. Right seamless moves are always attractive, and so, here are some ways to help you show your energy to the world.

Be mindful of every pace: Being conscious of how you move makes you slow, but this is a good advantage. Slowing down your steps will help you to understand so much about how your system works.

We will force every step we make when some parts of your body become painful to move. In such situations, we are often taught that if a part of the body is quite hard to move, to get out of it, it is best to move fast.

But this method will not result in majestic motion, and neither is it okay to move briskly.

Nevertheless, the best and sensible approach here is to be mindful of our body while in motion. In order words, slow down and be careful.

The secret to greater mobility is to be conscious; all other tips for moving are based on this single method.

Use Your Hips for power: The amount of energy flowing from the hips is enormous and glaring. The human body's gravitational pull is a few centimeters beneath the belly button. It puts the hips and butt just above and below.

The faster from this stage, you can start the movement; the more effective the movements will be as you move with less unnecessary motion. The hips have the body's power sources.

Follow the Direction of your Eyes: Use your eyes to trace the direction of your movement, and you will feel much steadier.

There's a sophisticated natural reaction known as the vestibulo-ocular reflex, which links the eyes to the whole body. Simply put, the brain is biologically programmed to trace your eye movements while and the entire body is programmed to follow your heart.

The whole body must meet the eyes. This is a universal truth utilized in Judo and any martial arts that: "the body moves in the direction of the head."

Squatting is a practical example of the body which follows the eyes in a movement. Also, if you would like an excellent spinal posture to keep your body standing and high, you must look directly at your front. When you are looking down, the muscle fibers in your head and the rest of your vertebrae will contract easily, contributing to a hostile stance.

Be mindful of Weight Transfer for Quick Stamina: checking your weight is important when you are trying to balance yourself out of a handstand or when you are about to trip and fall.

You must learn how to be mindful of your body weight from the moment you start moving to when you stop. This becomes easier when we know our center of gravity.

Carrying your weight properly is the start of a steady and guided movement Attempt this practice: keep your weight equally divided between the two legs; Then leap to your right instantly; Move over to the middle and pause for a brief moment after which you jump to the left. Try this again for both sides, shift carefully this time, keeping track of how your weight is moving.

Breathe Deeply for Quick Energy and Confidence: You will not have to chant any Buddhist meditation like "Om" or something, but certainly easy breathing is useful.

Most people forget to breathe – fortunately, we're mindlessly doing that, else people would be dying now and then.

People mindlessly hold their breath when moving, and this will quickly diminish one's energy. The body can mentally prepare itself when making a motion that needs some energy, although you don't do it intentionally.

Anxiety is often associated with breathing. When people are very anxious, they subconsciously hold their breaths. Therefore, you are prone to get frustrated easily if you move around without paying attention to how you breathe.

Bad breathing produces anxiousness, suspense, and lousy motion is caused by unmediated stress. Breathing slowly and purposefully contributes to steady and systematic movement.

Conclusion

What have you gained reading this book? Have you noticed the area that hits you the most?

If you have not gained anything yet, I suggest you read again, and this time, be more intimate with the book and passionate about getting something out of it. You need to get it right once and for all!

Emotional eating is not something that does not occur frequently. To state the fact, we have all done it at some point in our lives. And there is even the tendency that you will be tempted to eat in the coming weeks emotionally. We all can fall quickly to emotional eating. This is because most, if not all the situations we encounter are beyond our control. All we can do to these situations is to react or respond to it.

Everyone is vulnerable to emotional eating. As a result, we should not take it as something new or rather unusual. Instead, we should consider it as a behavior that we can live without. Living without this behavior can be challenging, sometimes due to its uncontrollable nature. While we consider the struggle of overcoming it, we should nevertheless, look at the other side of the table. If we do not overcome it, what are the things we are likely to face?

Eating in response to emotion works a great deal of harm to people. A study recently conducted found that emotional eating does not actually reduce stress. Instead, it increases emotional distress by igniting a strong sense of guilt after an emotional eating period. This is among the various detrimental effects of emotional eating.

Emotional eating features compulsion, and as a result, people often give up trying to fight it whenever the uncontrollable urge comes. Those that try not to fall for it are prone to exhibiting unusual behaviors such as trembling, shaking, nausea, and sometimes even begin to experience negative emotions. In other words, overcoming emotional eating can be hard, but living with it is harder. The adverse effects cover the psychological, social, and physical aspects.

In a bid to demystify emotional eating and proffer ways around the habitual behavior, this book comes in handy for that very purpose. This book has exhaustively discussed the theory of emotional eating as well as terms and concepts that are related to it. It has offered explanations that are reader-friendly and easy to understand, while also giving practical and useful tips and steps to overcoming each terminology discussed.

Lastly, the book should be your everyday companion. Read, digest the content, and apply it in your daily life. The triggers of emotional eating can come at any time. So, it is essential to be ready at all times. I hope this book has developed the mindset for change in you. Building a healthy lifestyle by making conscious efforts to control your eating habits and creating a healthy diet plan for yourself will go a long way in creating a successful life. And this book will do just that!

www.ingramcontent.com/pod-product-compliance
Lightning Source LLC
Chambersburg PA
CBHW070710250726
48662CB00001B/351